Adventures of Mom and Daughter YOGA

Rochelle Katzman

BALBOA
PRESS
A DIVISION OF HAY HOUSE

Balboa Press books may be ordered through booksellers or by contacting:

Balboa Press
A Division of Hay House
1663 Liberty Drive
Bloomington, IN 47403
www.balboapress.com
1 (877) 407-4847

Because of the dynamic nature of the Internet, any web addresses or links contained in
this book may have changed since publication and may no longer be valid. The views
expressed in this work are solely those of the author and do not necessarily reflect the views
of the publisher, and the publisher hereby disclaims any responsibility for them.

The author of this book does not dispense medical advice or prescribe the use of any technique
as a form of treatment for physical, emotional, or medical problems without the advice of a
physician, either directly or indirectly. The intent of the author is only to offer information
of a general nature to help you in your quest for emotional and spiritual well-being. In the
event you use any of the information in this book for yourself, which is your constitutional
right, the author and the publisher assume no responsibility for your actions.

Any people depicted in stock imagery provided by Thinkstock are models,
and such images are being used for illustrative purposes only.
Certain stock imagery © Thinkstock.

Printed in the United States of America.

ISBN: 978-1-4525-8407-2 (sc)
ISBN: 978-1-4525-8408-9 (e)

Library of Congress Control Number: 2013918405

Balboa Press rev. date: 12/19/2013

Table of Contents

♥ This book belongs to

Mom   _____

Daughter   _____

_____

♥

_____

♥ Dedication ♥

This book is dedicated to my best friend, Karen Block Katzman, my beautiful mom.

There are yoga books that use professional models photographed in yoga postures by the ocean or in other breathtaking locations. I wanted to present real moms and daughters in real homes doing yoga. This book was created to show all moms and daughters everywhere, no matter how hectic their lives are, that they can also do yoga and enjoy quality time together.

The moms and daughters photographed in this book are my students, friends, and good neighbors. I loved watching them grow together through my yoga program giving them an enriched, joyful experience. I hope you enjoy the photos too!

♡ Rochelle

The people in this book are actual mothers and daughters photographed in real homes.

Breathing helps you focus and keeps you calm. Take three deep breaths through your nose before you begin each story. After each posture always inhale and exhale through your nose.

As the stories are being read, sit in easy pose in between postures (cross-legged). See example below.

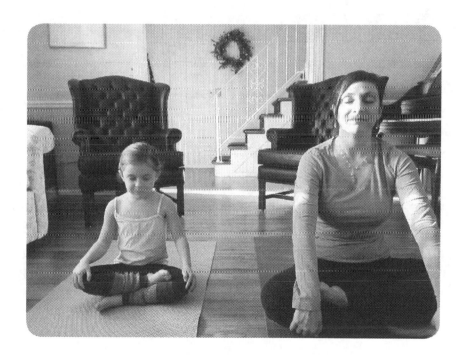

Don't forget to breathe
before each story.
♡ Rochelle

RELAX

At the end of each story, allow yourself time to relax. Lie on your back with your palms facing up. Close your eyes. (3-11 minutes)

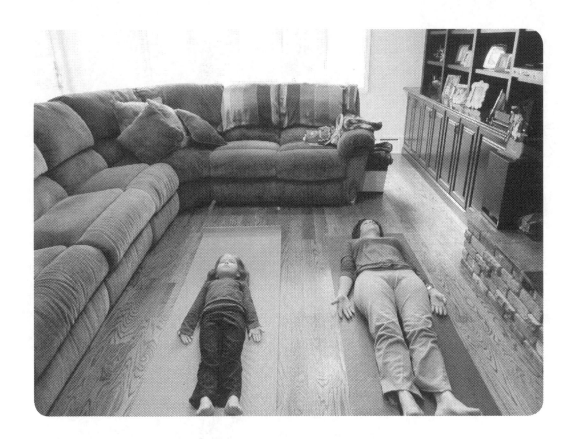

So Relaxing !
♥ Rochelle

Mom and daughter awake one Saturday morning, and they stretch.

Stretch

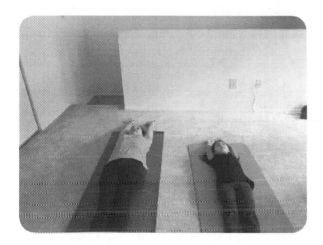

Move your arms and legs all around.
(1-3 minutes)

They decide to go hiking in the Catskill Mountains in Upstate New York. They travel by car until they reach the bottom of a mountain. Then they get out of the car and look at the majestic scenery.

Sufi Grind

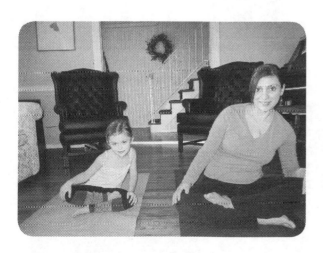

Sit in easy pose (cross-legged). Place hands on knees and move your spine all around, then change direction.
(1-3 minutes in each direction)

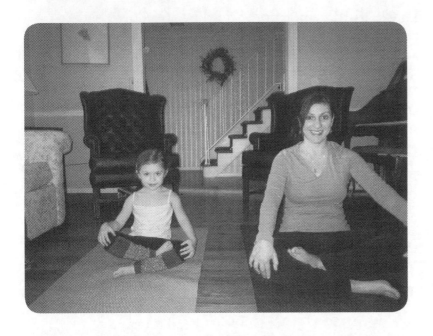

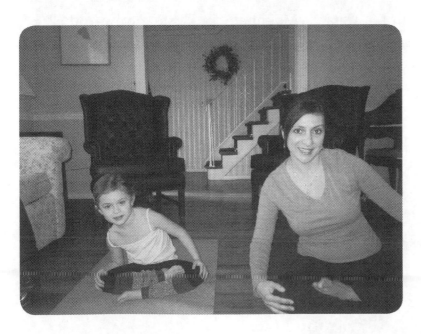

They look to the left and to the right.

Spinal Twist

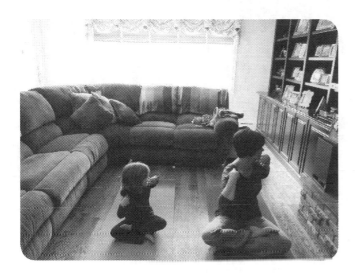

Place your hands on your shoulders and twist from left to right. (1-3 minutes)

Mom and daughter see something very strange. They see a cat and a cow together hanging out.

Cat and Cow

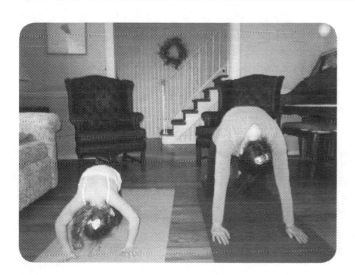

On your hands and knees, inhale and arch your spine up and head down. Exhale and arch your spine down and head up. (1-3 minutes)

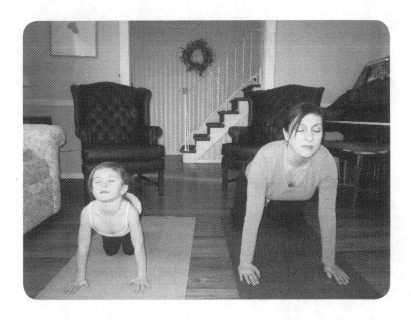

They see the cat and the cow climbing the mountain. They decide to climb the mountain too.

Downward Facing Dog (Triangle Pose)

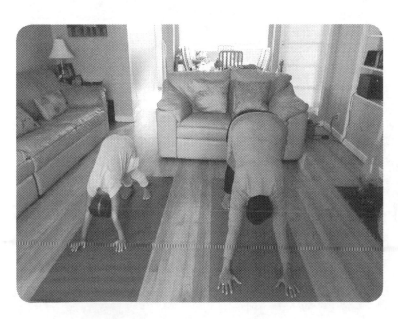

Looks like a mountain. Place the palms of your hands and the soles of your feet flat on the ground. Feet are approximately hip-width apart. (1-2 minutes)

They run up the mountain.

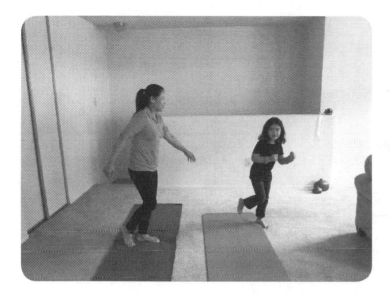

Run all around the room.
(1-3 minutes)

Mom thinks it is such a beautiful day that she feels they should stop and enjoy the sun.

Cobra Pose

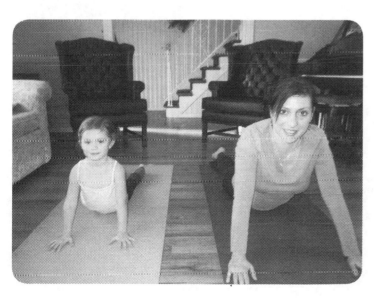

Lie on your stomach. Place your hands under your shoulders and your palms flat on the ground. Then push your chest and arms up until your arms are straight. If you are not flexible, you may place your elbows on the ground. Look up, and don't forget to inhale and exhale. (1-3 minutes)

By that time the cat and cow are gone. Mom and daughter are getting very tired. They decide to rest.

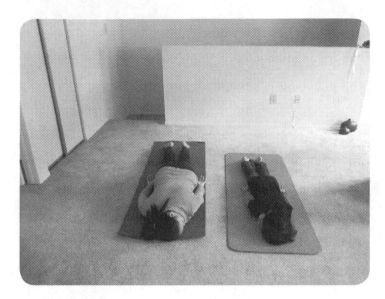

Lie on your stomach with mom's head facing daughter's head. Place your arms by your sides with palms facing up. Close your eyes. (1-3 minutes)

When they awaken, it is time to head down the mountain.

Downward Facing Dog (Triangle Pose)

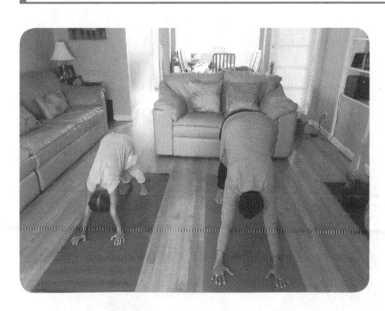

Looks like a mountain. Place the palms of your hands and the soles of your feet flat on the ground. Feet are approximately hip-width apart. (1-2 minutes)

All of a sudden, they reach a rainforest, and it starts raining very hard.

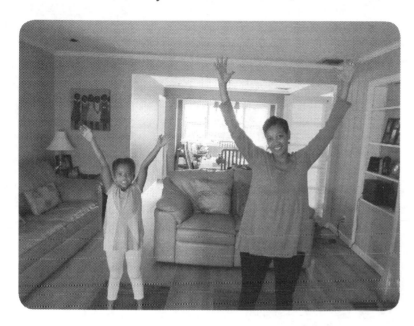

Act like a rainstorm. Stand and shake arms really fast. (1-3 minutes)

They speedily run the rest of the way down the mountain.

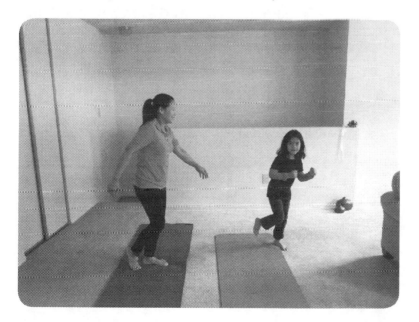

Run all around the room. (1-3 minutes)

While they are going down, they continue to see beautifully colored trees.

Partner Tree Pose

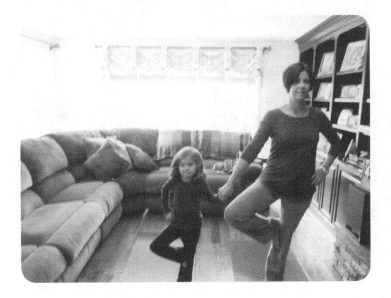

Stand on one leg with the other leg bent touching your knee or thigh. Mom and daughter hold on to each other. Change legs. It helps with balance if you find a spot and focus on it. (1-3 minutes each side)

When they finally reach the bottom of the mountain, they look back and thank the mountain for a wonderful day.

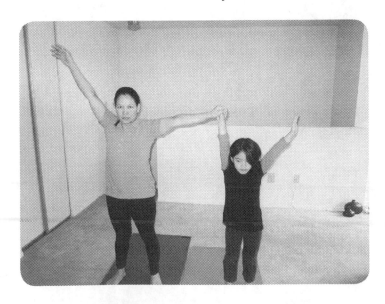

Mom and daughter raise arms up in the air while standing. (1 minute)

Then mom and daughter hug.

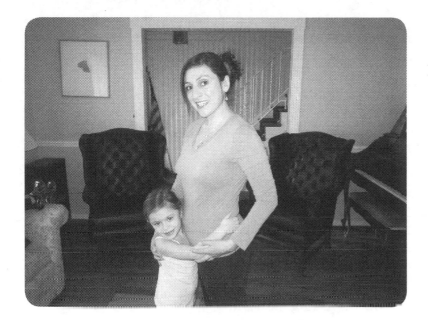

Hug

Give your mom a
huge hug!
♡ Rochelle

Mom and daughter return from hiking in Upstate New York. When they get home, mom looks through the mail and sees an invitation. She opens the invitation. It says that she and one guest are invited to meet a prince and princess at a party at Buckingham Palace in London. The party is in two weeks. Naturally, mom chooses to take her daughter. Mom decides they should take a cruise ship to London, so they pack their bags and go to the ship. Once the ship is in the ocean, they see a lot of waves.

Partner Rowboat

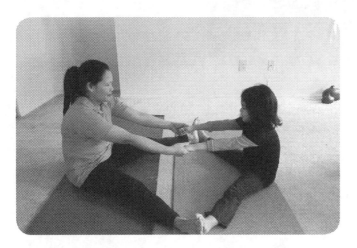

Mom and daughter get into a partner pose where the mom is seated and her legs are open really wide. The daughter either matches the mom and their feet touch or the daughter spreads her legs enough to place her feet on her mom's calves. Their hands connect, and they move back and forth, really stretching the spine. Move like a strong wave. (1-3 minutes)

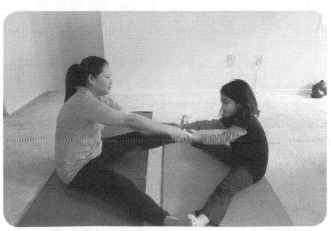

Stay in the same pose. Instead of moving back and forth, mom and daughter move in big circles. (1-3 minutes)

The ocean is so beautiful. They see miles and miles of water and birds are overhead.

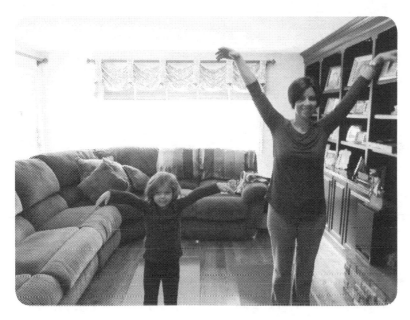

Stand up and fly like a bird around the room. Raise your arms very high. (1-3 minutes)

All of a sudden the sky becomes very gray. All they can see are dark clouds. Then it starts to rain.

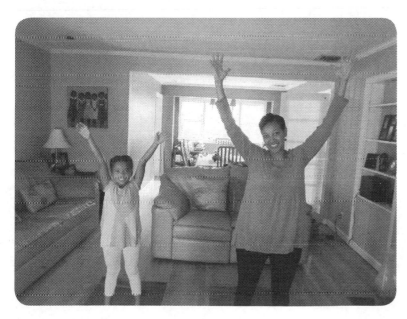

Act like a rainstorm. Stand and shake arms really fast. (1-3 minutes)

The ship rocks back and forth and the waves are now huge.

Partner Rowboat

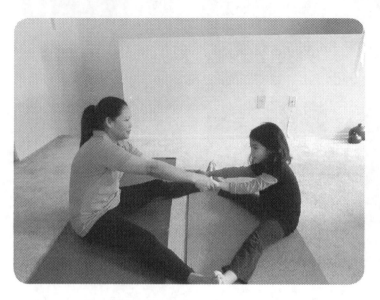

Go back to the partner pose where the mom is seated and her legs are open really wide. The daughter either matches the mom and their feet touch or the daughter spreads her legs enough to place her feet on her mom's calves. Connect hands and move in big circles, faster than the last time. Move like a big wave. (1-3 minutes)

Mom and daughter think that if they go inside the ship and lie down for a nap, the rain soon will stop, and it will become sunny.

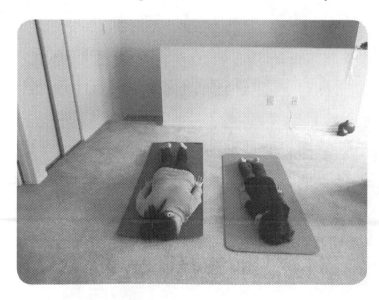

Lie on your stomach with mom's head facing daughter's head. Place your arms by your sides with palms facing up. Close your eyes. (1-3 minutes)

Sure enough, they are right! When they wake-up it is sunny outside. They think that this is the perfect time to sit by the pool and relax, but they see a problem. There is only one unoccupied chair by the pool. They decide to take turns sitting on the chair.

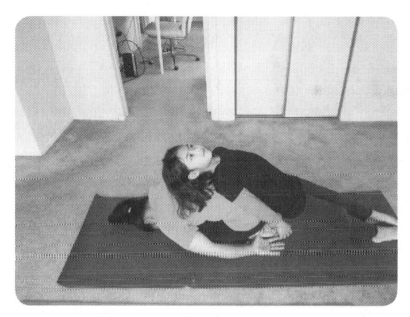

Mom sits in baby pose, sitting on her heels with her stomach on the ground and her arms by her side with the palms facing up. Daughter lies over the mom. Both their backs connect, and the daughter stretches her feet out. Then they change positions. The mom adjusts according to her daughter's size. (1-3 minutes each person)

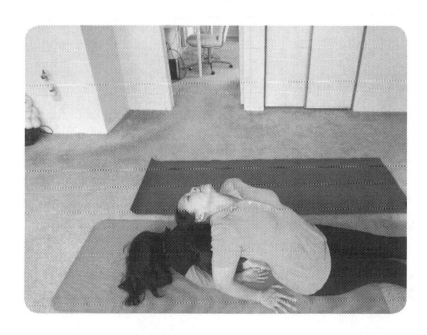

Finally, they see land and mountains.

Downward Facing Dog (Triangle Pose)

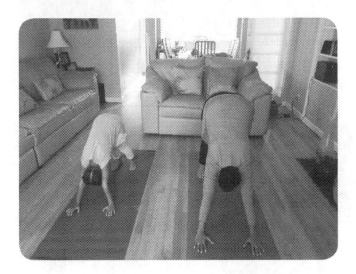

Looks like a mountain. Place the palms of your hands and the soles of your feet flat on the ground. Feet are approximately hip-width apart. (1-2 minutes)

They arrive at the dock in London, England. They pack their bags, get off the boat, and look all around.

Sufi Grind

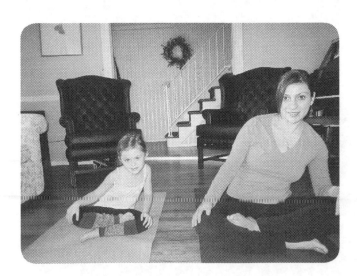

Sit in easy pose (cross-legged). Place hands on knees and move your spine all around, then change direction. (1-3 minutes each direction)

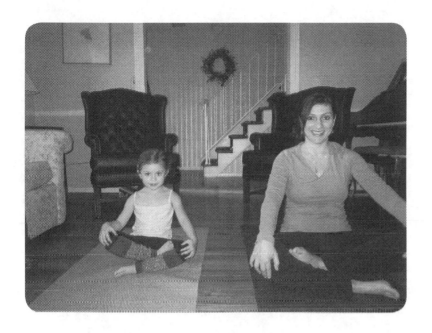

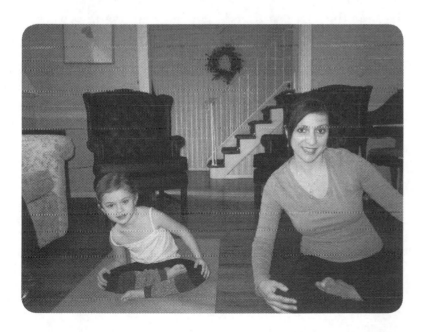

Then they look from left to right.

Spinal Twist

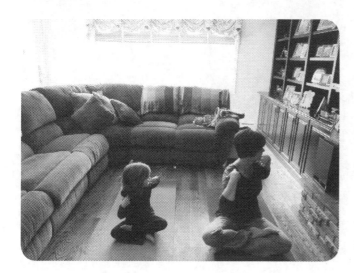

Place your hands on your shoulders and twist from left to right. (1-3 minutes)

They think London is incredible, and they are so excited to meet a prince and princess. They find a taxi to take them to Buckingham Palace. They tell the taxi driver to go quickly because they can't wait to get there. The taxi driver drives under a bridge.

Bridge Pose

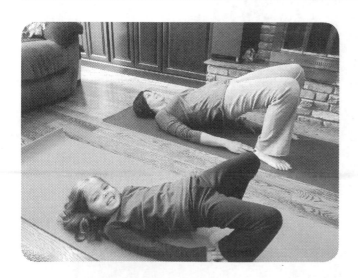

Lie on your back with your legs bent close to your body and your head on the floor. Place your hands on your ankles. Lift up above the ground. Keep breathing. (1-3 minutes)

At last, they arrive at the palace. They get out of the cab and wave good-bye to their very nice taxi driver. Mom and daughter are so excited that they hug!

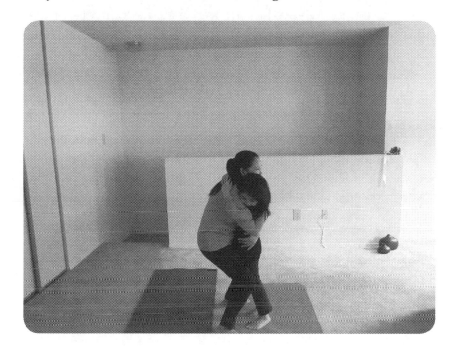

Hug

Buckingham palace is
so beautiful.

♡ Rochelle

Mom and daughter walk into the palace, where they are told they are to meet a prince and princess in the ballroom for the party. The ballroom is up the steps, down the hall to the left, and then through the second door on the right at the end of the hallway. They then turn left followed by a quick right. The ballroom is the last door on the left.

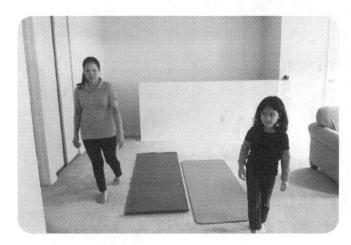

Walk all around the room.
(1-3 minutes)

They enter the big ballroom, and they see a prince and princess. They walk up to them and bow.

Yoga Bow

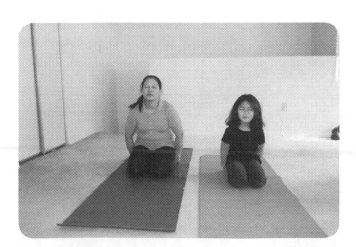

Sit on your heels. Inhale and stretch your spine up. Exhale forward bringing your forehead to the ground. Have your third eye point touch the ground.

Your third eye point is the point in between your eyebrows.
(1-3 minutes)

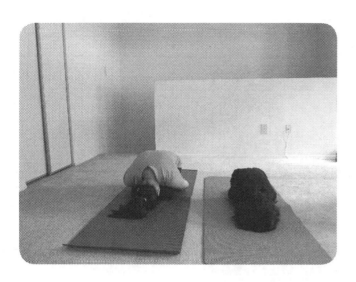

When they finish greeting them—the princess is wearing a beautiful pink gown that goes to the floor, her hair is down, and she is wearing diamond earrings and a beautiful necklace—mom and daughter walk to the center of the room and look all around.

Sufi Grind

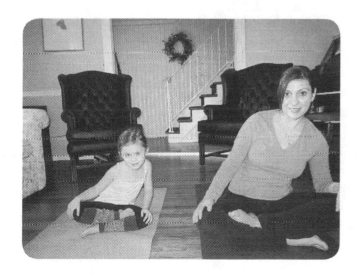

Sit in easy pose (cross-legged). Place hands on knees and move your spine all around, then change direction. (1-3 minutes each direction)

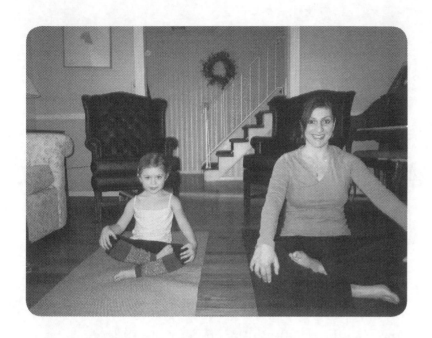

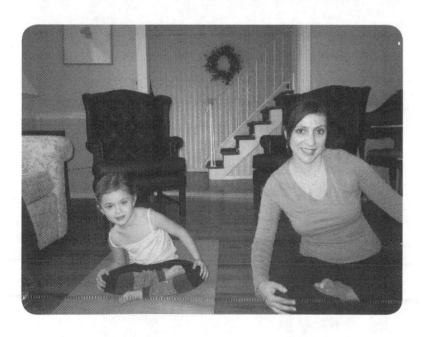

Then they look from left to right.

Spinal Twist

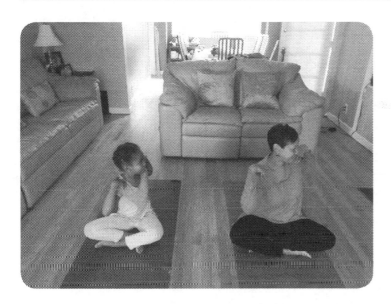

Place your hands on your shoulders, and twist from left to right. (1-3 minutes)

Everyone looks lovely. There must be one hundred people in the room, and everyone is dancing.

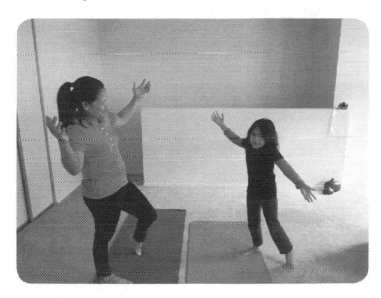

Dance and don't forget to have fun! (1-3 minutes)

They are dancing and dancing. Before they know it, it is the middle of the night. They approach the prince and princess and say, "Good night." They bow again.

Yoga Bow

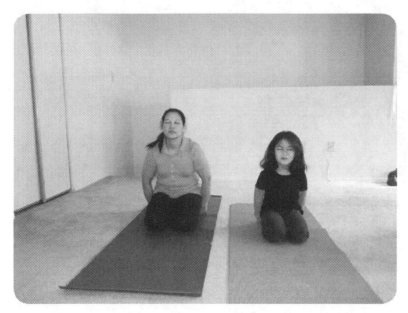

Sit on your heels. Inhale and stretch your spine up. Exhale forward bringing your forehead to the ground. Have your third eye point touch the ground. Your third eye point is the point in between your eyebrows. (1-3 minutes)

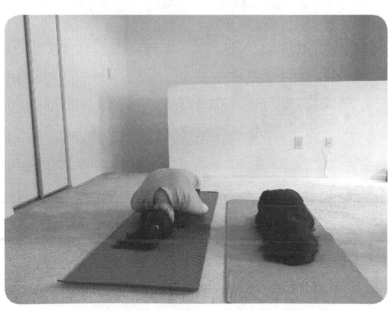

Then they go to one of the bedrooms in the palace and sleep.

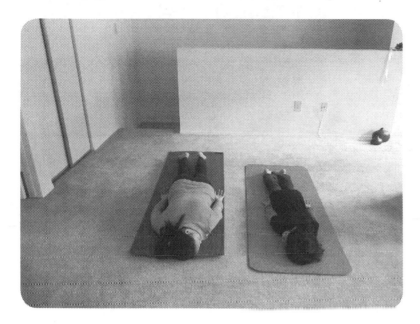

Lie on your stomach with mom's head facing the daughter's head. Place your arms by your side with palms facing up. Close your eyes. (1-3 minutes)

They wake up the next morning and stretch.

Cat Stretch

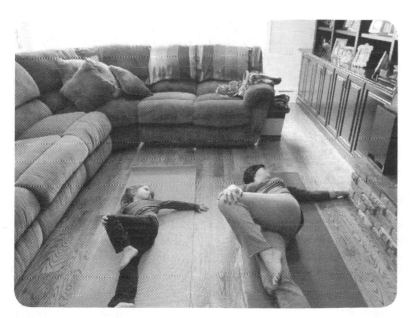

Lie on your back, bend your left knee. Put left leg over right and place your left arm out to the side. Then change to the other leg. (1-3 minutes each side)

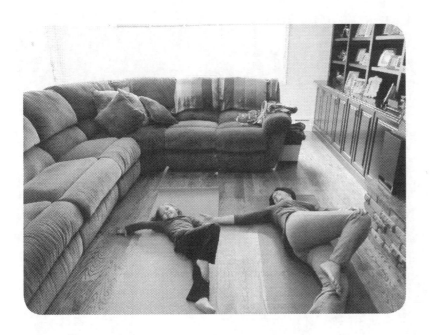

They decide that, since they are already in Europe, they should stay for a few days and visit different countries. Today they decide to go to Switzerland to visit the huge mountains of the Swiss Alps. They travel to the airport and get on a plane to go to Switzerland.

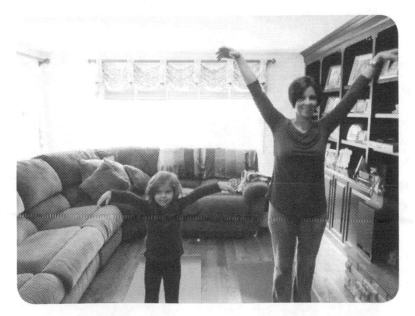

Stand up and fly like a bird all around the room. Raise your arms very high. (1-3 minutes)

They land in Switzerland and travel to the Alps. The mountains are huge!

Downward Facing Dog (Triangle Pose)

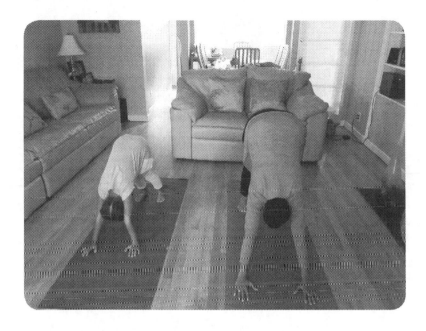

Looks like a mountain. Place the palms of your hands and the soles of your feet flat on the ground. Feet are approximately hip-width apart. (1-2 minutes)

They begin walking up the mountain.

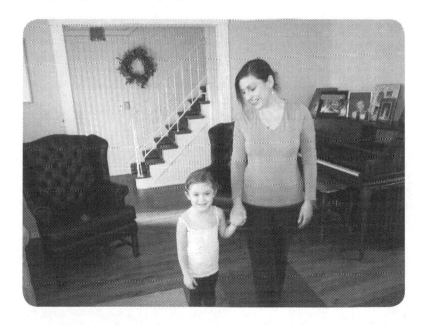

Walk around the room holding hands. (1-3 minutes)

They see beautiful trees.

Partner Tree Pose

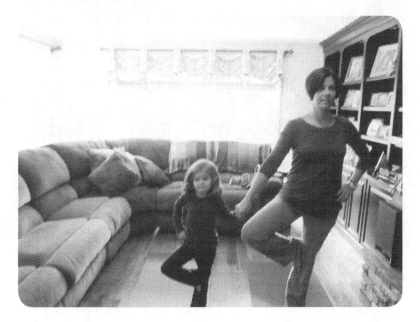

Stand on one leg with the other leg bent touching your knee or thigh. Mom and daughter hold on to each other. Change legs. It helps with balance if you find a spot and focus on it. (1-3 minutes each side)

While they walk to the top of the mountain, it gets very windy.

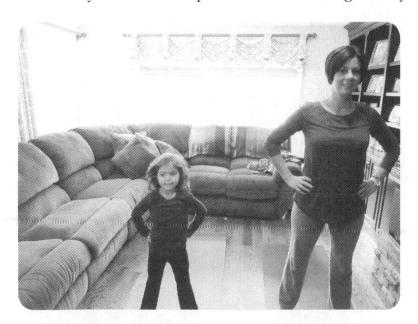

Stand hip-width apart with hands on hips and move your spine in big circles making noise that sounds like wind. (1-3 minutes)

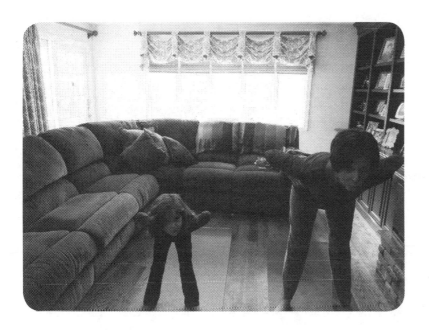

It is so windy that they decide to go back down the mountain. When they are walking down the mountain, they see many beautiful butterflies.

Butterfly

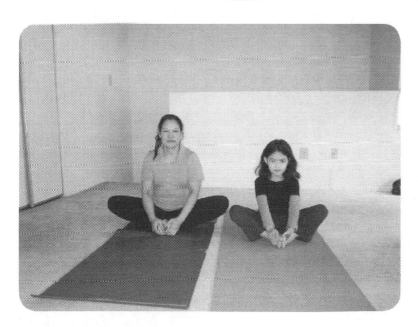

Sit in easy pose with your feet together, knees bent, and move legs back and forth. Place hands on your feet. (1-3 minutes)

They watch the butterflies fly and land on the ground. On the ground are some seeds from the trees. Mom and daughter think it is a great idea to plant the seeds in the ground. This will be a symbol for years to come that they were here. They begin planting the seeds.

Seed Pose

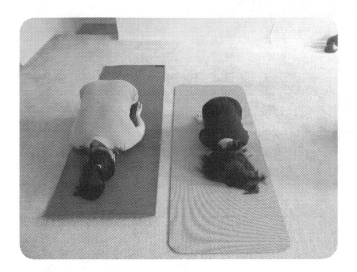

Begin in baby pose, on your heels with your stomach and head facing the ground. Bring arms back. (1 minute)

They watch the seeds begin to grow and the trees get bigger and bigger.

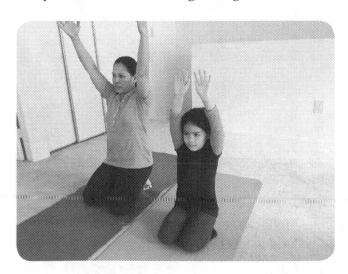

Stretch your arms up and get bigger and bigger by slowly standing up.

And even bigger!

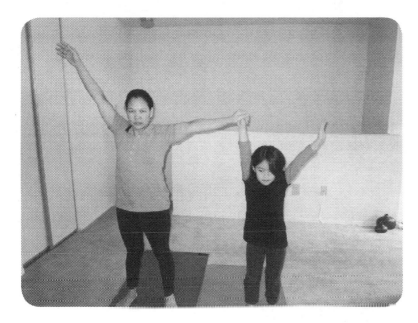

Once standing, mom and daughter grab hands and reach toward the sky. (1 minute)

Mom and daughter are really happy. They continue to walk to the bottom of the mountain and they hug.

Then they drive to the airport and their European adventure continues ...

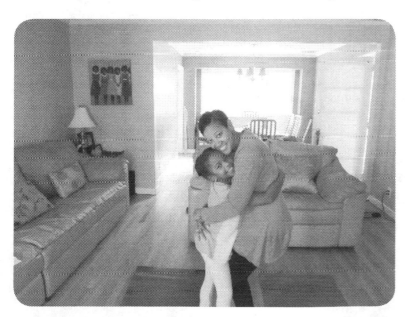

Hug

Mom and daughter are at the airport deciding where they should go next. The daughter always wanted to see a beautiful castle in Ireland, so they go on their iPad and look up Irish castles. The most beautiful castle they can find is outside Dublin, Ireland. They quickly get on a plane to Dublin.

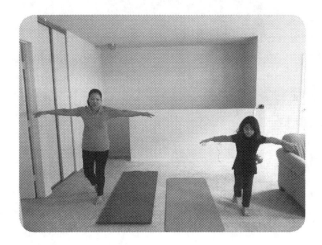

Stand up and fly like a bird around the room. Raise your arms very high. (1-3 minutes)

When they arrive in Dublin, they get in a cab and ask to go to the castle.

Spinal Flex

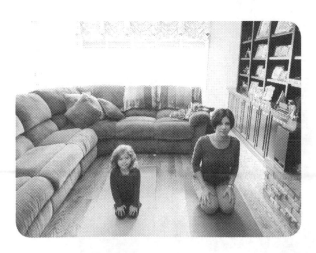

Sit on your heels in rock pose. Move your spine front and back as fast as you can with your hands on your knees. Looks like a bumpy cab ride. (1-3 minutes)

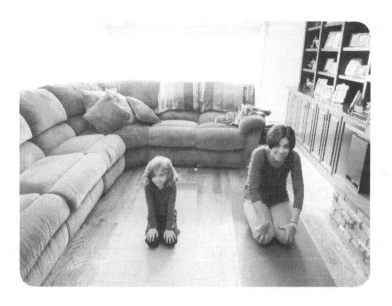

The countryside of Ireland is so beautiful. Can you believe that mom and daughter pass a lot of cats and cows?

Cat and Cow

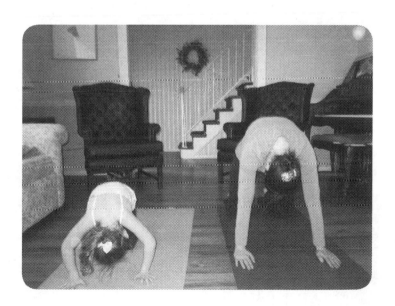

On your hands and knees inhale and arch your spine up and head down. Exhale and arch your spine down and head up. (1-3 minutes)

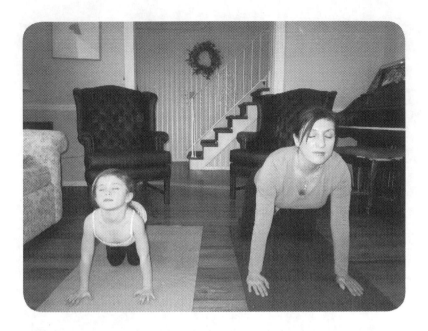

They pass people on bicycles too.

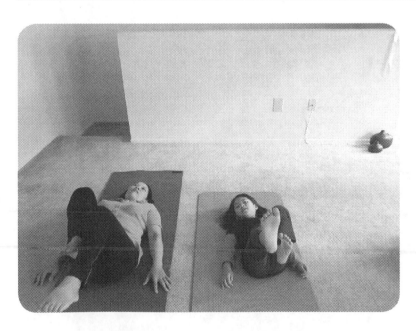

Lie on your back. Put your legs in the air and move them in fast circles like a fast bicycle. (2-3 minutes)

And they pass beautiful windmills.

Windmill

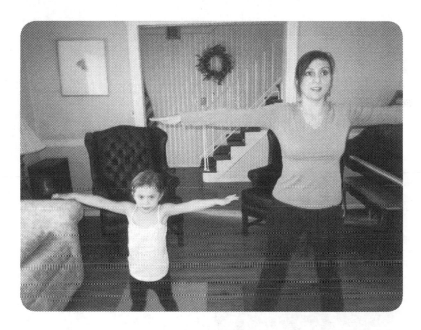

Stand with your legs apart. Put your arms out parallel to the floor. Bend and touch your left hand to your right foot. Then stand straight. Bend and touch your right hand to your left foot. Look up in the air. (1-3 minutes)

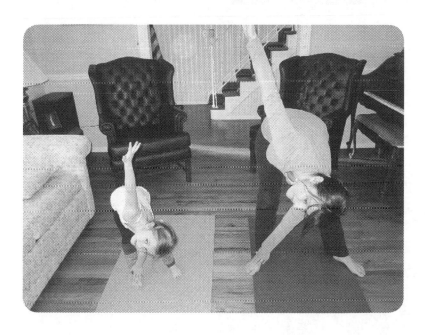

Finally, they reach the huge castle. They've never seen anything so magnificent. They get out of the cab and look all around.

Sufi Grind

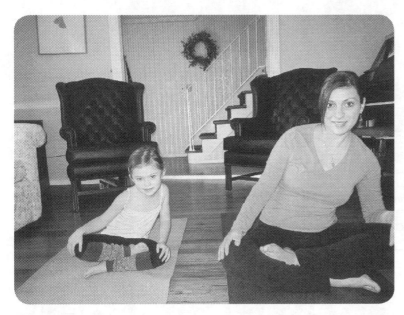

Sit in easy pose (cross-legged). Place hands on knees and move your spine all around, then change direction. (1-3 minutes each direction)

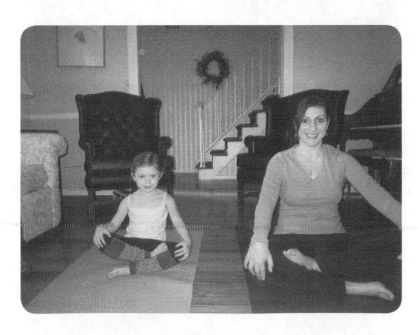

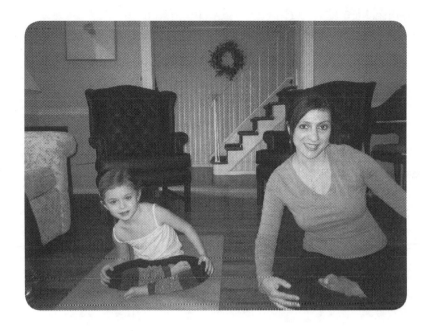

Then they look from left to right.

Spinal Twist

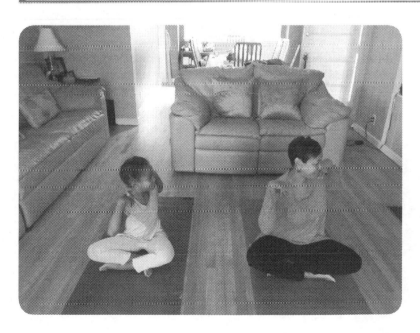

Place your hands on your shoulders and twist from left to right. (1-3 minutes)

Mom and daughter are so excited that they do the yoga twist!

Yoga Twist

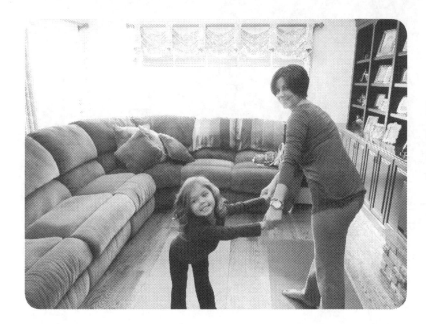

Mom and daughter face each other, hold hands and twist in opposite directions. (1-3 minutes)

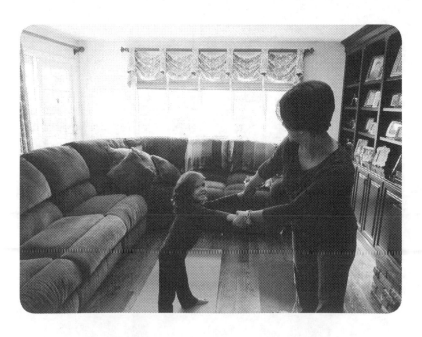

They stand outside the castle realizing that they can't go in because there is a huge body of water (a moat) around the castle. Luckily, there is a rowboat.

Partner Rowboat

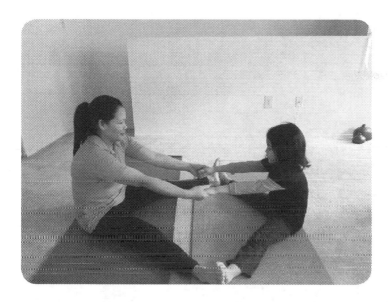

Mom and daughter get into a partner pose where the mom is seated and her legs are open really wide. The daughter either matches the mom and their feet touch or the daughter spreads her legs enough to place her feet on her mom's calves. Their hands connect, and they move back and forth really stretching the spine. (1-3 minutes)

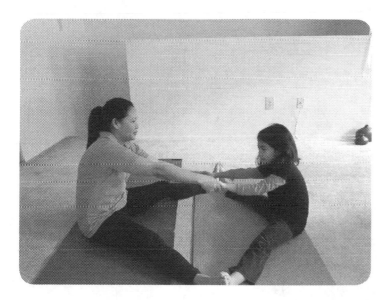

Stay in the same pose, but move spine around in big circles. (1-3 minutes)

They get out of the boat and enter the castle. A butler meets them at the front door and tells them to walk around for a while, after which he will serve them tea in the garden. The mom and daughter start to walk.

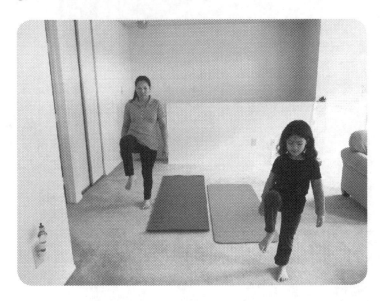

Stand up and walk all around the room taking very big steps, raising your knees high. (1-3 minutes)

The castle is so beautiful. There are so many statues.

Archer Pose (Warrior Pose)

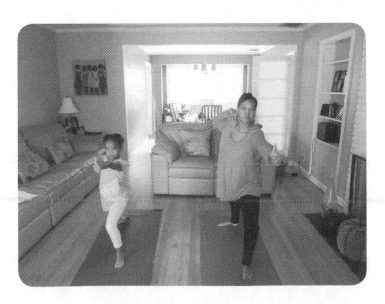

Stand and place your left foot in front facing forward and your right foot in the back facing the side. Bend your left leg slightly. Bring your left arm out straight and your right arm bent by your shoulder. Stare straight ahead. Looks like a statue. Change legs. (1-3 minutes each side)

Some of the rooms have clouds painted on the ceilings.

Camel Pose (Looks like a Cloud)

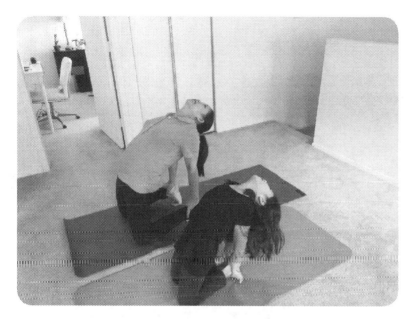

Sit on your knees, straighten your spine, and lean back. Grab your ankles or heels. Adjust yourself according to your flexibility. Push the heart center upward. (1-3 minutes)

Mom and daughter get tired so they go into one of the bedrooms and lie down.

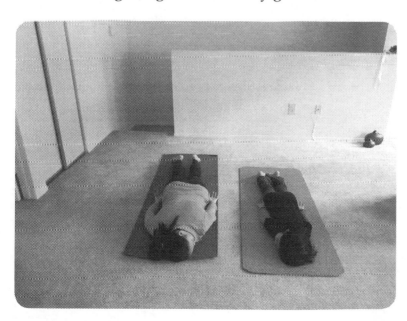

Lie on your stomach with mom's head facing the daughter's head. Place your arms by your sides with palms facing up. Close your eyes. (1-3 minutes)

When they awaken, they are very hungry. They decide to go outside to the garden and drink tea. While they are outside it starts to rain.

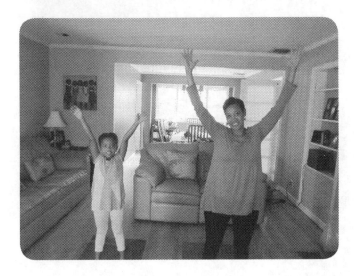

Act like a rainstorm. Stand and shake arms really fast. (1-3 minutes)

Then, all of a sudden it stops raining, and they see the most beautiful rainbow. It is the prettiest rainbow they have ever seen. In front of the rainbow there's a magnificent butterfly.

Butterfly

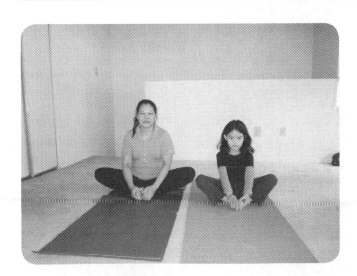

Sit in easy pose with your feet together, knees bent and move legs back and forth. Place hands on your feet. (1-3 minutes)

Near the butterfly there stands a tiny leprechaun, and next to the leprechaun is a huge pot of gold. They bow to the leprechaun, and he gives them the pot of gold.

Yoga Bow

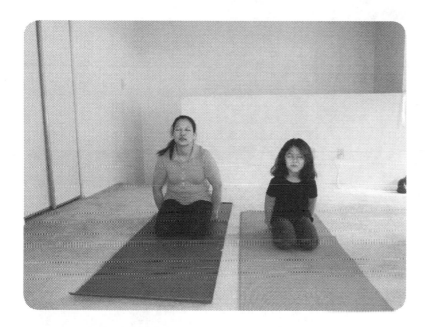

Sit on your heels. Inhale and stretch your spine up. Exhale forward bringing your forehead to the ground. Have your third eye point touch the ground. Your third eye point is the point in between your eyebrows. (1-3 minutes)

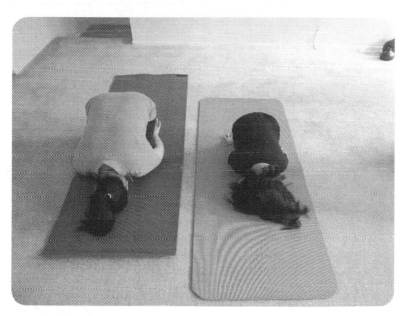

They are so excited! Mom and daughter thank the leprechaun. They can't believe that they have all this gold. They are so happy that the mom and daughter hug.

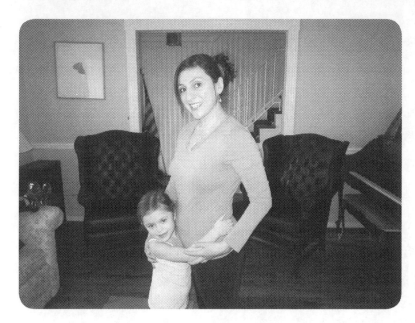

Hug

Give your daughter
a huge hug!
♥ Rochelle

With the big pot of gold in their hands, they now have a lot more money than they ever imagined. They decide that they will donate a lot of the money to charity, but they will keep a little of the gold to finish traveling through Europe. Mom and daughter now wish to leave Ireland. The South of France would be perfect. Since they have all this money, they decide they will find a yacht and sail to the South of France. The first thing they need to do is find a limousine to drive them to the harbor. The butler at the castle arranges for a limousine and a driver. They get into the limousine.

Spinal Flex

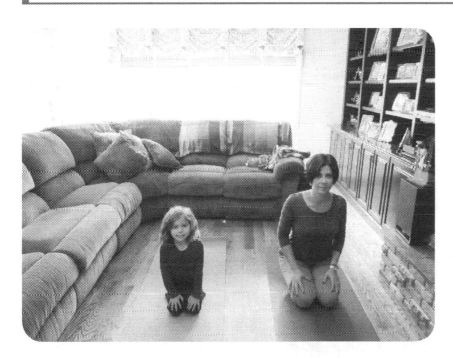

Sit on your heels in rock pose. Move your spine front and back as fast as you can with your hands on your knees. Looks like a bumpy limousine ride. (1-3 minutes)

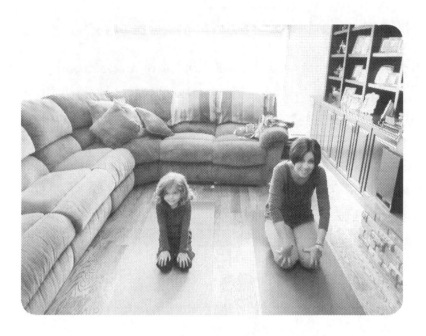

To get to the harbor they have to go over large hills.

Downward Facing Dog (Triangle Pose)

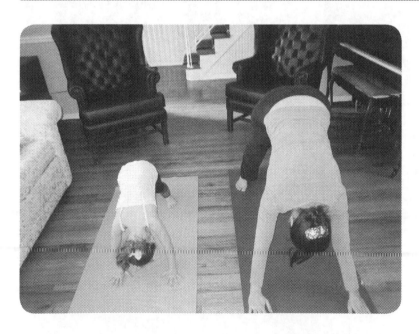

Looks like a mountain. Place the palms of your hands and the soles of your feet flat on the ground. Feet are approximately hip-width apart. (1-2 minutes)

They also have to go under bridges.

Bridge Pose

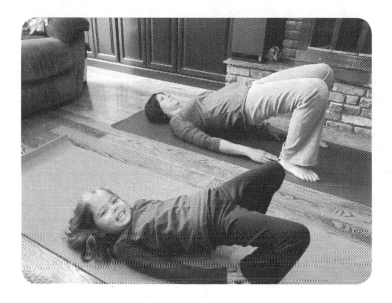

Lie on your back with your legs bent close to your body and your head on the floor. Place your hands on your ankles. Lift up above the ground. Keep breathing. (1-3 minutes)

Finally, they reach the harbor. They find the perfect yacht to take them to the South of France. They quickly make the arrangements and board.

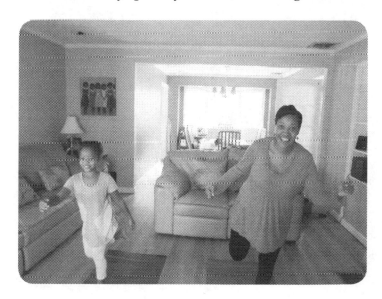

Run all around the room. (1-3 minutes)

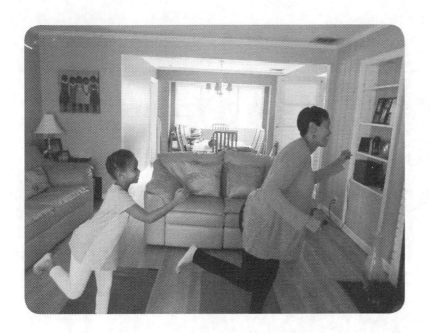

It is so magnificent. The inside has beautiful wood on the walls and chandeliers hanging down from the ceilings. When the yacht leaves the harbor, the first thing they decide to do is swim in the pool.

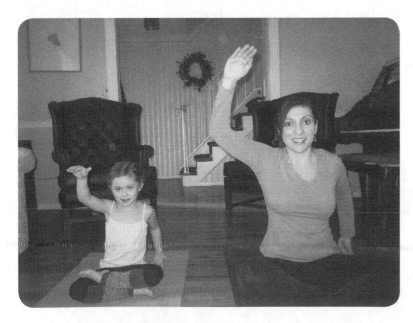

Sit in easy pose and move your arms over your head as if you are swimming. (1-3 minutes)

When they are finished swimming they lie out by the pool.

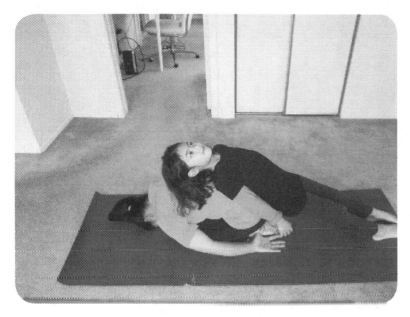

Mom sits in baby pose, sitting on her heels with her stomach on the ground and her arms by her side with the palms facing up. Daughter lies over the mom. Both their backs connect and the daughter stretches her feet out. Then they change positions. The mom adjusts according to her daughter's size. (1-3 minutes each person)

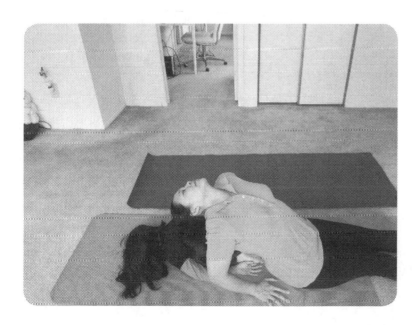

Meanwhile, they look at the ocean and see a small island. On the island are sea lions.

Sea Lion

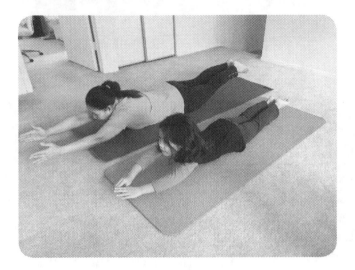

Lie on stomach with calves and feet raised. Place your arms forward and raise your chest. Make sea lion noises. (1-3 minutes)

They run to the railing to look at the sea lions. Then they look at the ocean and see a lot of fish.

Fish Pose

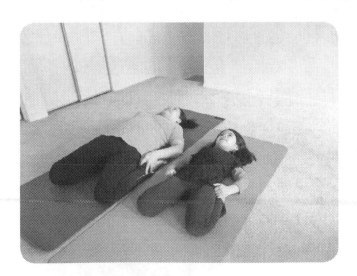

Lie on back. Bend your knees and place your feet by your hips. (1-3 minutes)

Mom yells, "Look, look!" She sees penguins by the island.

Rocking Bow Pose

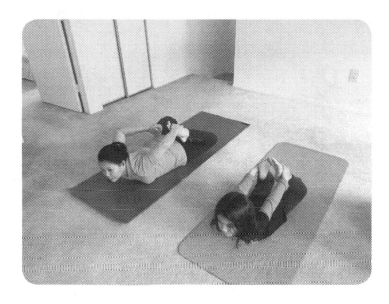

Lie on stomach, grab ankles, and raise your bent legs and upper body. Begin to rock back and forth. Pretend you're a penguin. (1 minute)

Mom and daughter are having so much fun. Then all of a sudden the waves get really rough.

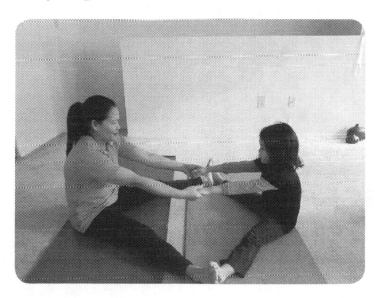

Mom and daughter get into a partner pose where the mom is seated and her legs are open really wide. The daughter either matches the mom and their feet touch or the daughter spreads her legs enough to place her feet on her mom's calves. Their hands connect, and they move back and forth really stretching the spine. (1-3 minutes)

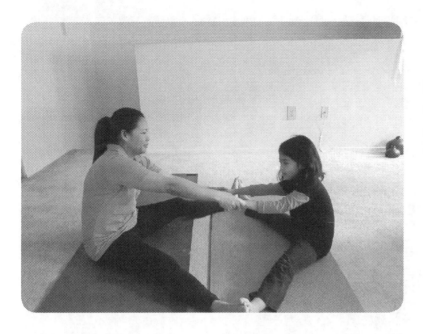

Stay in the same pose, but circle your arms and spine around. Move like a big wave. (1-3 minutes)

The birds in the sky are making loud noises and are flying away.

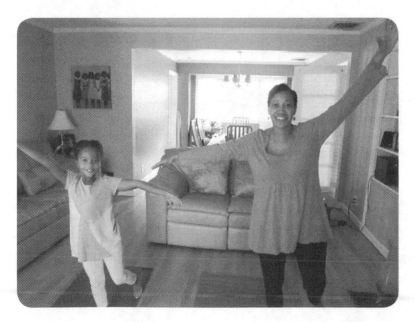

Stand up and fly like a bird all around the room. Raise your arms very high. (1-3 minutes)

Of course, it starts to rain.

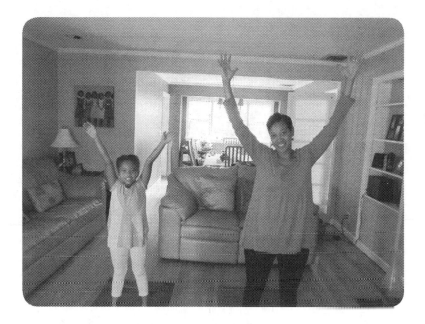

Act like a rainstorm. Stand and shake arms really fast. (1-3 minutes)

It gets very windy.

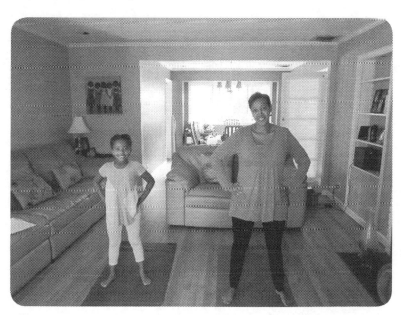

Stand hip-width apart with hands on hips and move your spine in big circles making a noise that sounds like wind. (1-3 minutes)

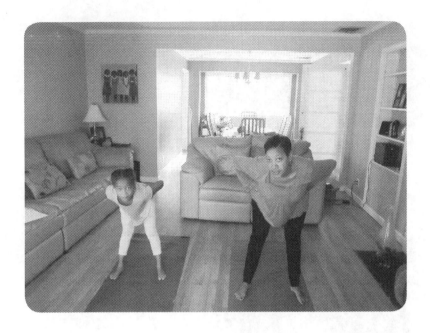

Mom and daughter decide to go inside and get a massage at the spa on the ship.

Neck Rolls

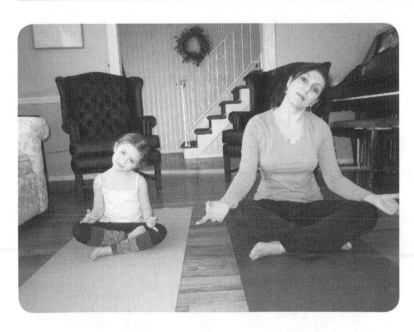

Sit in easy pose, and move your neck in circles changing direction. (1-3 minutes each side)

Shoulder Shrugs

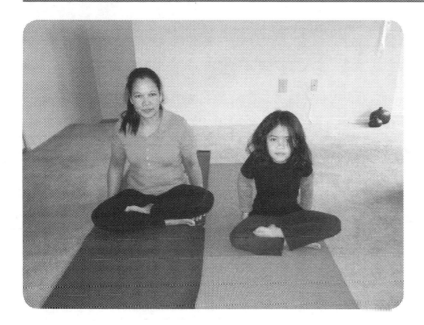

Move shoulders up and down. (1-3 minutes)

The spa is so beautiful. There are candles all around.

Shoulder Stand (Candle)

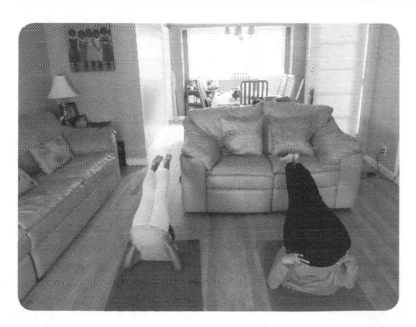

Lie on back and push your legs up, head and shoulders on the ground. Your hands can rest on your lower back. This looks like a candle. (1-2 minutes)

All of this makes them very sleepy. They are so tired. They leave the spa and go to their cabin and lie down to sleep.

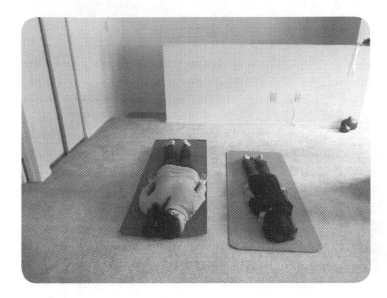

Lie on your stomach with mom's head facing daughter's head. Place your arms by your sides with palms facing up. Close your eyes. (1-3 minutes)

When they awaken, they look outside. It no longer raining, and they have arrived in the South of France. They are so excited that they grab their bags, get off the yacht, and walk to the beach. They are so happy that they hug.

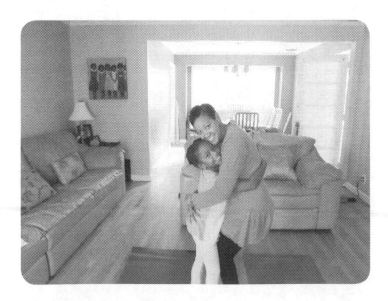

Hug

Mom and daughter excitedly arrive in the South of France. The first thing they need to do is check into a hotel. They walk, and walk, and walk all around to find a nice hotel.

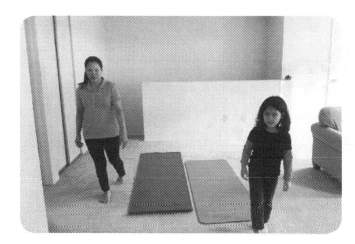

Walk all around the room.
(1-3 minutes)

Finally they find a chateau which was converted into a hotel. They walk into this beautiful chateau and the owner, Monsieur Jacques, greets them. He says, "Bonjour" which means "Hello" in English. Mom and daughter give him a warm greeting.

Yoga Bow

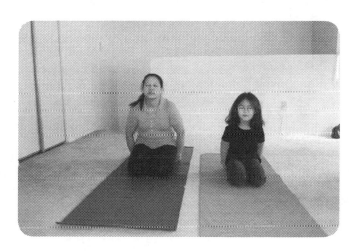

Sit on your heels. Inhale and stretch your spine up. Exhale forward bringing your forehead to the ground. Have your third eye point touch the ground. Your third eye point is the point in between your eyebrows. (1-3 minutes)

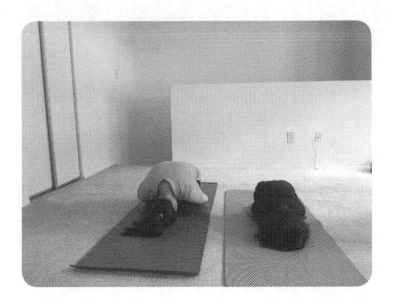

Monsieur Jacques leads them into the lobby of the chateau which has beautiful chandeliers and huge windows that overlook the sea. Mom and daughter look all around.

Sufi Grind

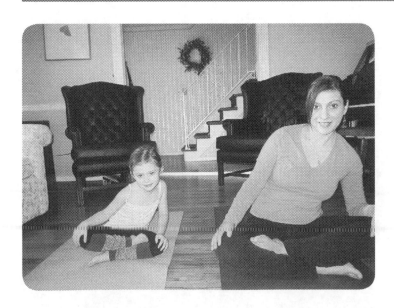

Sit in easy pose (cross-legged). Place hands on knees and move your spine all around, then change direction. (1-3 minutes each direction)

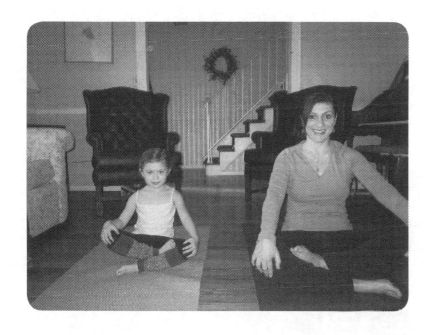

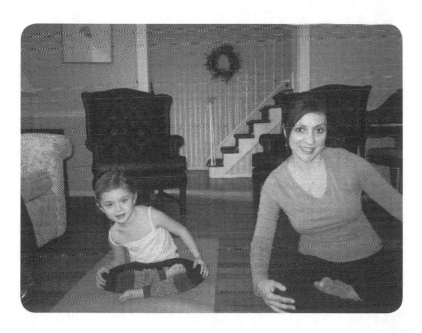

Then look from left to right.

Spinal Twist

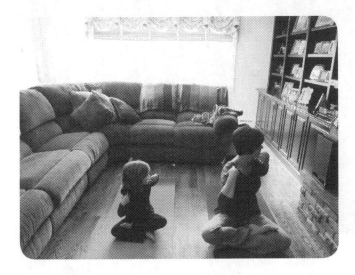

Place your hands on your shoulders and twist from left to right. (1-3 minutes)

Monsieur Jacques shows them to their room and says that they may borrow two bicycles to ride to an area on the beach that is private and beautiful. They drop their luggage in their room and borrow the bicycles.

Bicycle Pose

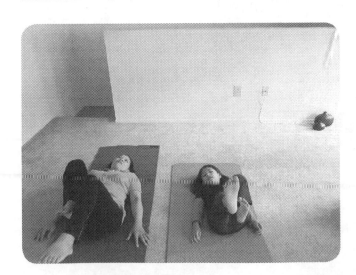

Lie on your back. Put your legs in the air and move them in fast circles like a fast bicycle. (1-3 minutes)

They ride their bicycles down a beautiful path. At the end is the magnificent beach that Monsieur Jacques told them about. It is truly breathtaking. They drop everything and decide to go for a swim.

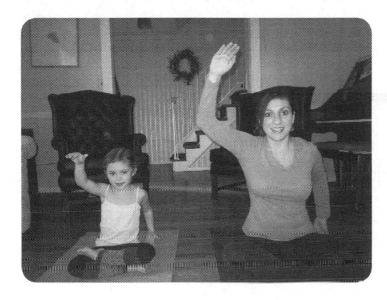

Sit in easy pose and move your arms as if you are swimming. (1-3 minutes)

The sea is so clear. They can see a lot of little fish.

Fish Pose

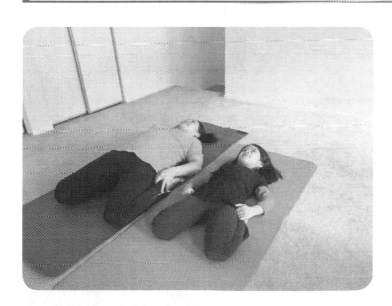

Lie on back. Bend your knees and place your feet by your hips. (1-3 minutes)

They even see sea lions far out in the distance.

Sea Lion

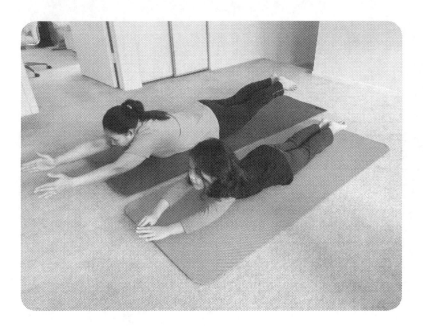

Lie on stomach with calves and feet raised. Place your arms forward and raise your chest. Make sea lion noises. (1-3 minutes)

Birds are flying all around.

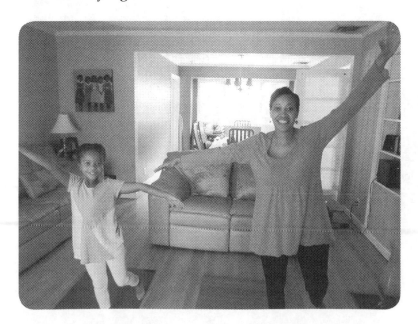

Stand up and fly like a bird around the room. Raise your arms very high. (1-3 minutes)

Mom decides they should meditate at the beach and do yoga poses.

Meditation Pose

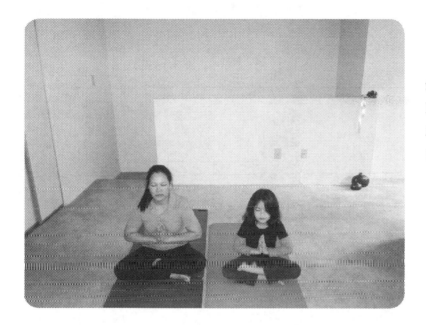

Sit in easy pose with your hands in prayer pose in front of your heart center. (1-3 minutes)

Sun Salutation Series

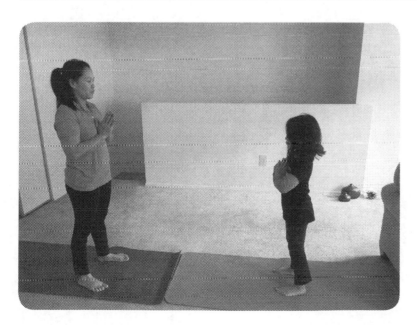

Mom and daughter arrange their mats facing each other.

Stand with hands in prayer pose at your heart center, facing each other with your eyes closed.

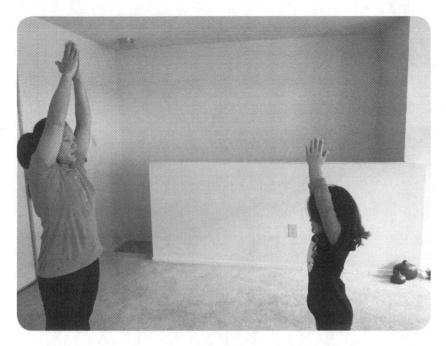

Move hands above your head in prayer pose.

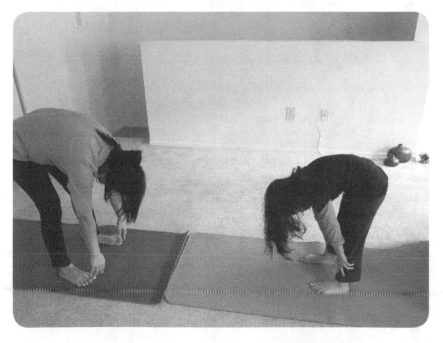

Bend down touching your toes.

Plank Pose

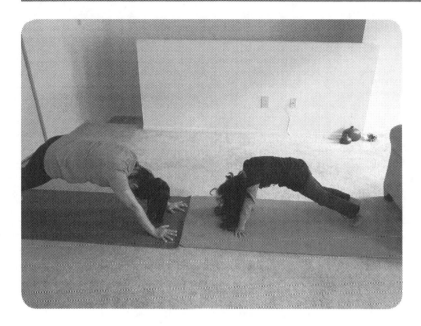

Place palms flat on the ground. Place your legs back. Push up and keep your body as straight as you can.

Cobra Pose

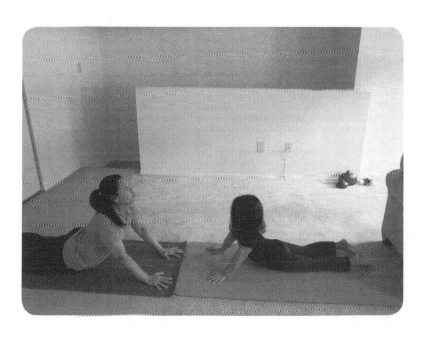

Lie on your stomach. Place your hands under your shoulders and your palms flat on the ground. Then push your chest and arms up until your arms are straight. If you're not flexible you may place your elbows on the ground. Look up and don't forget to inhale and exhale.

Downward Facing Dog (Triangle Pose)

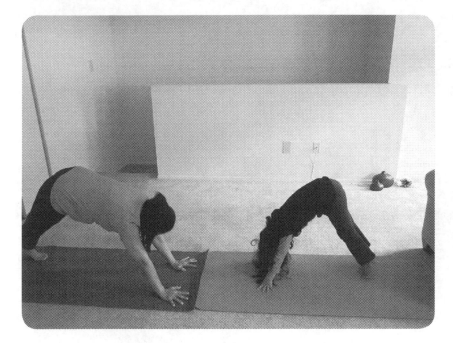

Place the palms of your hands and the soles of your feet flat on the ground. Feet are approximately hip-width apart.

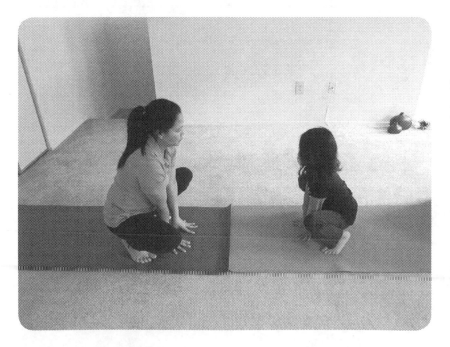

Squat down with your ankles touching and your hands on the ground.

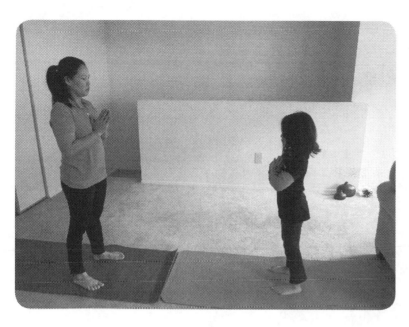

Stand with hands in prayer pose at your heart center.

Face each other throughout the Sun Salutation Series. Try to keep your eyes closed as much as possible. Repeat series 3-5 times.

The daughter's favorite posture is camel pose, so after sun salutation they do this pose.

Camel Pose

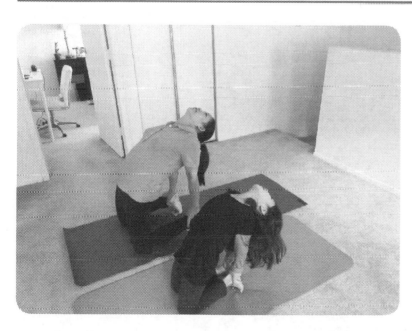

Sit on your knees, straighten your spine, and lean back. Grab your ankles or heels. Adjust yourself according to your flexibility. Push the heart center upward. (1-3 minutes)

And they rest.

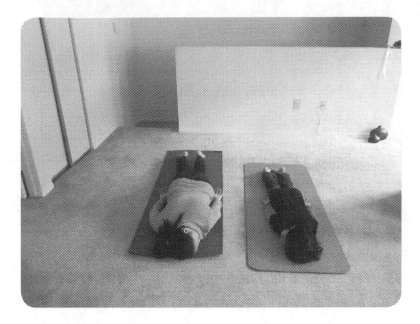

Lie on your stomach with mom's head facing the daughter's head. Place your arms by your sides with the palms facing up. Close your eyes. (1-3 minutes)

When they wake-up, they stretch.

Cat Stretch

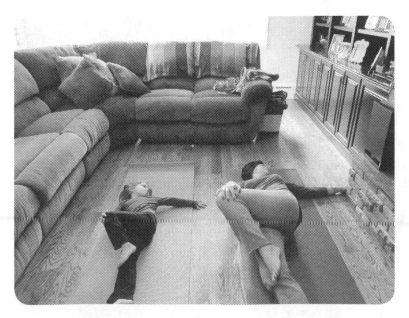

Lie on your back, bend your left knee. Put left leg over right and place your left arm out to the side. Then change to the other leg. (1-3 minutes each side)

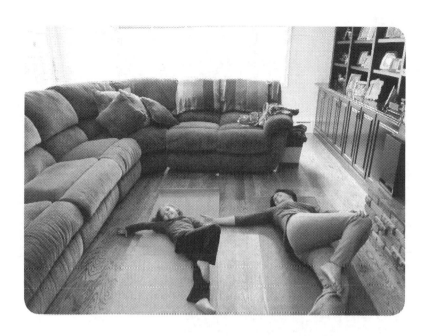

It is time to go back to the chateau. Instead of riding bicycles, they decide they should walk.

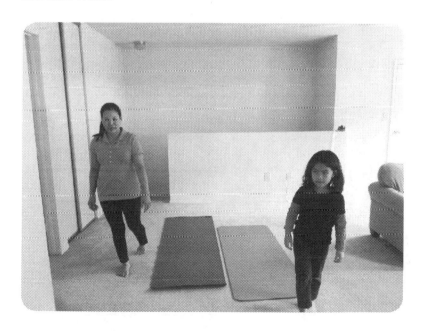

Stand up and walk all around the room. (1-3 minutes)

When they get back to their chateau they are so happy that they hug.

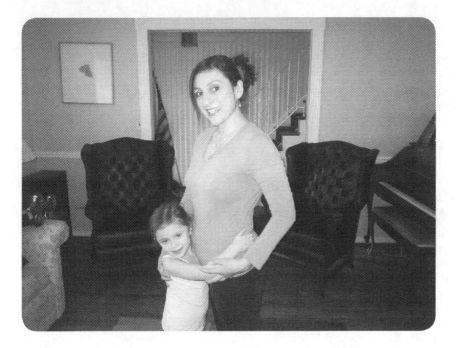

Hug

I love hugging my mom!
♡ Rochelle

Mom and daughter wake up in their beautiful chateau room in the South of France, and they stretch.

Stretch

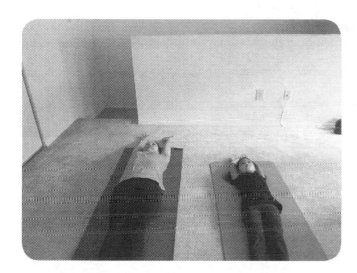

Move your arms and legs all around. (1-3 minutes)

Cat Stretch

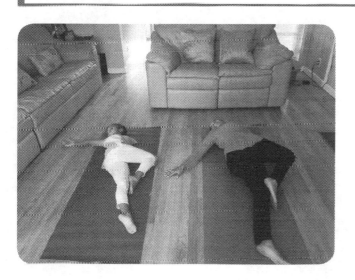

Lie on your back, bend your right knee. Put right leg over left and place your right arm out to the side. Then change to the other leg. (1-3 minutes each side)

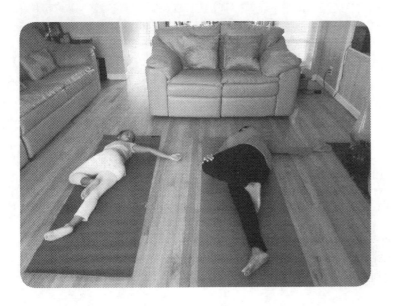

When they are fully awake they decide that they want to leave the South of France and go to Tuscany, Italy. They both always wanted to go to Tuscany. It is so beautiful there. They aren't in the mood to take a plane, and they think it will be fun to take a train. They go to the train station and get on a train to Tuscany.

Train

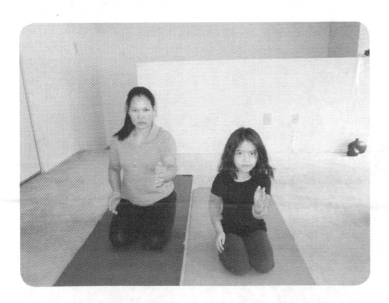

Sit in rock pose, on your heels and move your arms back and forth by your sides as fast as you can with elbows bent. Looks like a train. (1-3 minutes)

The train ride is lovely. The countryside of Italy is gorgeous. They pass windmills.

Windmill

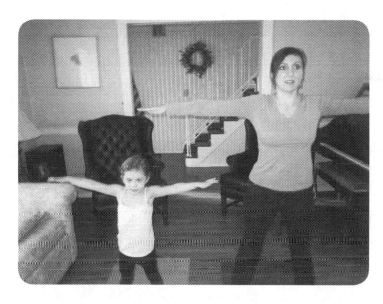

Stand with your legs apart. Put your arms out parallel to the floor. Bend and touch your left hand to your right foot. Then stand straight. Bend and touch your right hand to your left foot. Look up in the air. (1-3 minutes)

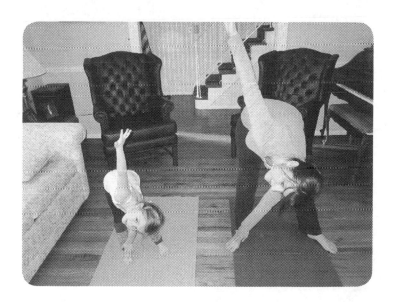

They pass many people on bicycles.

Bicycle Pose

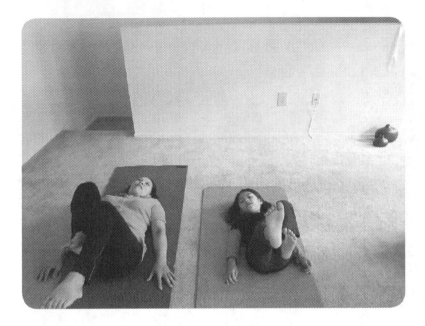

Lie on your back. Put your legs in the air and move them in fast circles like a fast bicycle. (2-3 minutes)

There are people slowly walking along the countryside.

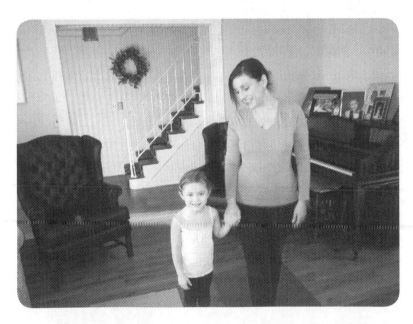

Stand up and walk around the room holding hands with your mom. (1-3 minutes)

Other people are jogging.

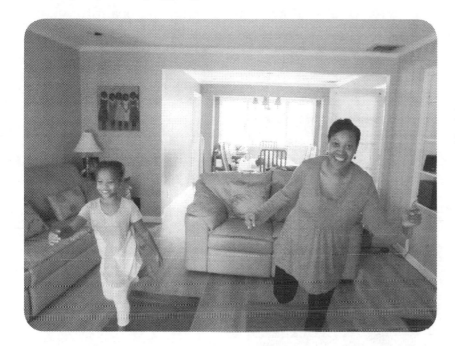

Run all around the room. (1-3 minutes)

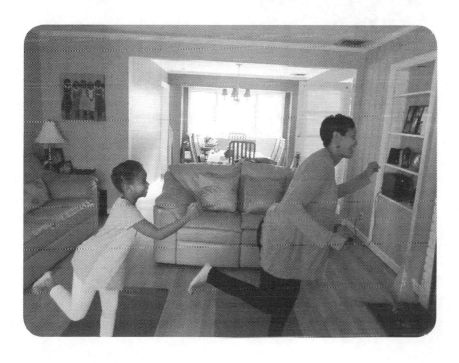

When the train stops and they arrive in the middle of Tuscany—it is so impressive. There are rolling hills and tall mountains, flowers all around, and beautiful villas. Mom and daughter are so happy. They look all around.

Sufi Grind

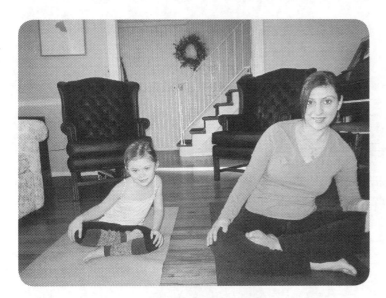

Sit in easy pose (cross-legged). Place hands on knees and move your spine all around, then change direction. (1-3 minutes each direction)

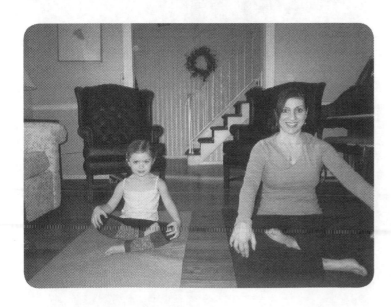

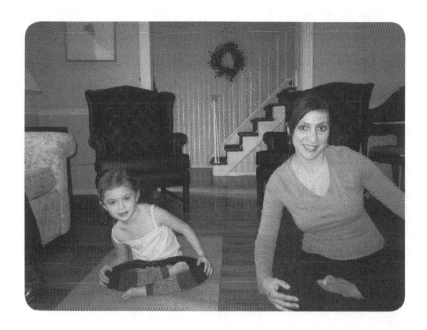

Then they look from left to right.

Spinal Twist

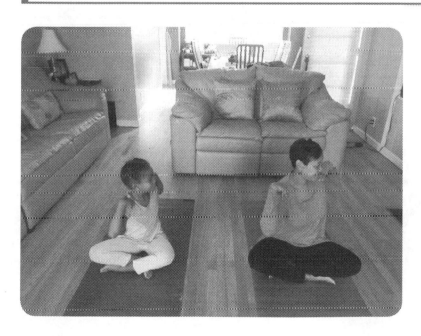

Place your hands on your shoulders and twist from left to right. (1-3 minutes)

They need to find a villa to stay in, so they walk, and walk, and walk.

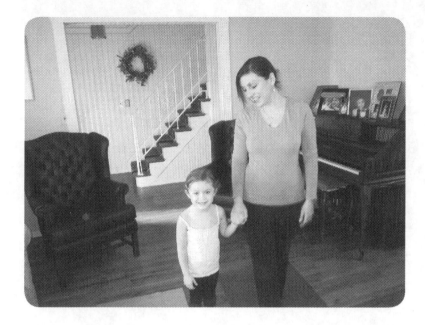

Stand up and walk around the room holding mom's hand. (1-3 minutes)

While they are walking, they see beautiful birds.

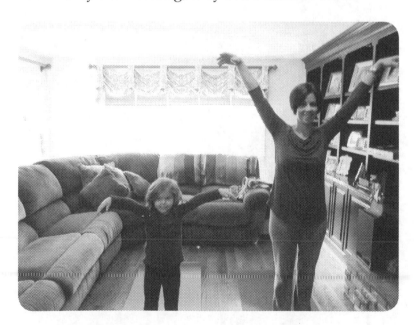

Stay standing and fly like a bird all around the room. Raise your arms very high. (1-3 minutes)

Finally, they see the most beautiful villa with a sign that reads, "Rooms for Rent." They walk into the villa, and it feels like home. They sit on a huge couch in the middle of the entrance hall and relax.

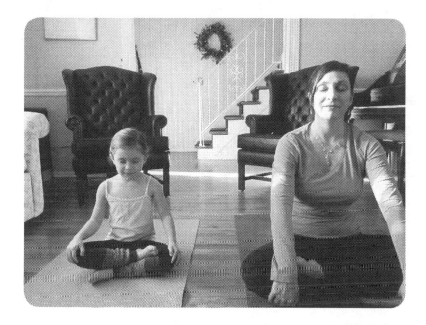

Inhale and exhale through your nose and take three deep breaths.

Neck Rolls

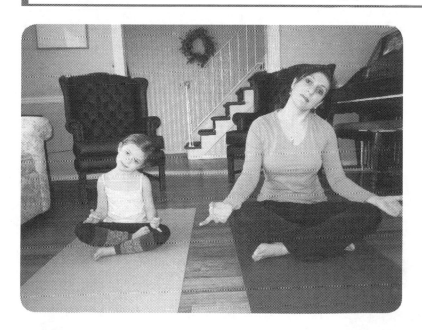

Sit in easy pose and move your neck in circles changing direction. (1-3 minutes each side)

Shoulder Shrugs

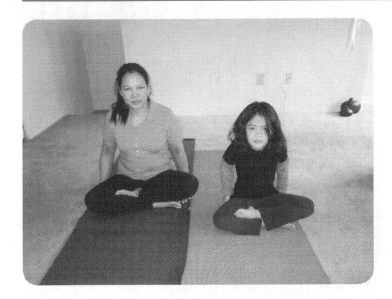

Move shoulders up and down. (1-3 minutes)

Just then a man named Antonio comes up to them and says that he is the owner of this Tuscan villa. They greet each other.

Yoga Bow

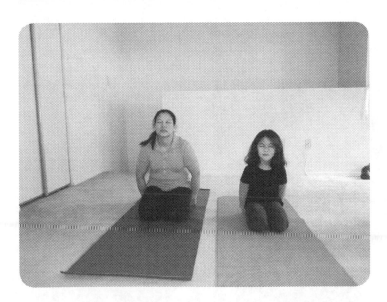

Sit on your heels. Inhale and stretch your spine up. Exhale forward bringing your forehead to the ground. Have your third eye point touch the ground. Your third eye point is the point in between your eyebrows. (1-3 minutes)

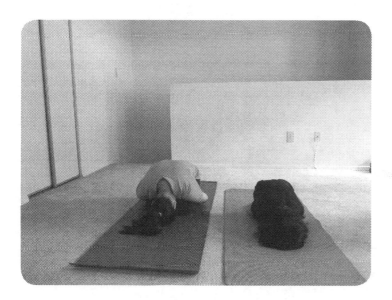

He tells them that he has one room left which overlooks the mountains of Tuscany. He shows them to their room. They look out the window and see the beautiful mountains.

Downward Facing Dog (Triangle Pose)

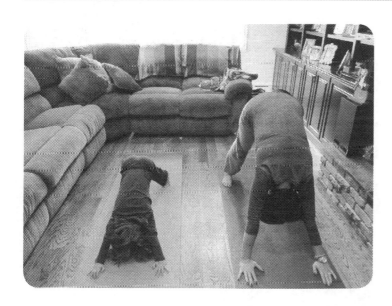

Looks like a mountain. Place the palms of your hands and the soles of your feet flat on the ground. Feet are approximately hip-width apart. (1-2 minutes)

There are also many trees.

Partner Tree Pose

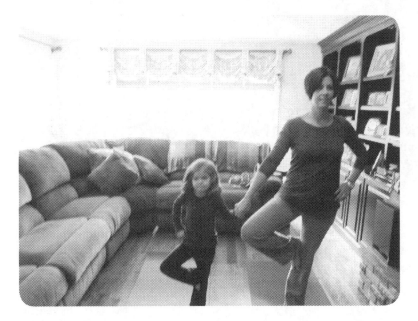

Stand on one leg with the other leg bent touching your knee or thigh. Mom and daughter hold on to each other. Change legs. It helps with balance if you find a spot and focus on it. (1-3 minutes each side)

Mom and daughter are so happy to be in Tuscany that they hug.

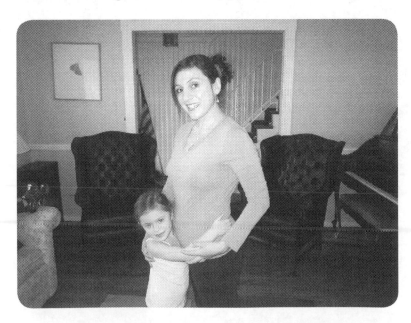

Hug

Mom and daughter wake up in their beautiful villa in Tuscany, and they stretch.

Stretch

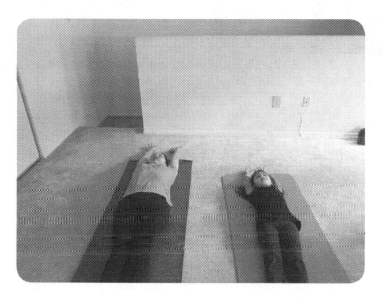

Move your arms and legs all around. (1-3 minutes)

Cat Stretch

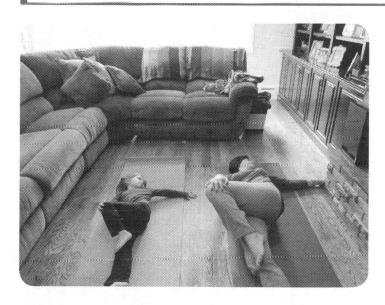

Lie on your back, bend your left knee. Put left leg over right and place your left arm out to the side. Then change to the other leg. (1-3 minutes each side)

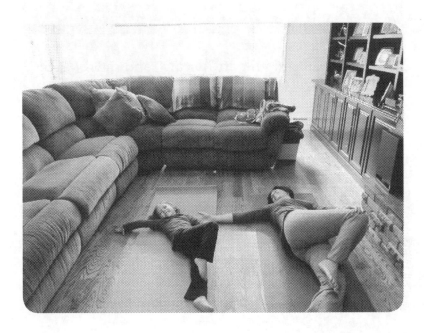

They get out of bed, open the window, and see that it is a sunny day. They welcome the sunlight into their room.

Sun Salutation Series

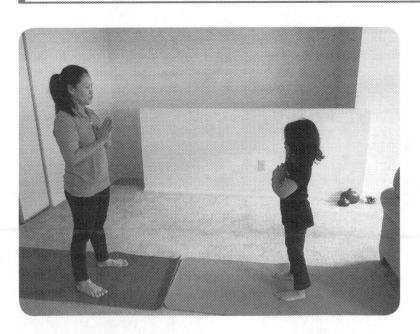

Mom and daughter arrange their mats facing each other.

Stand with hands in prayer pose at your heart center, facing each other with your eyes closed.

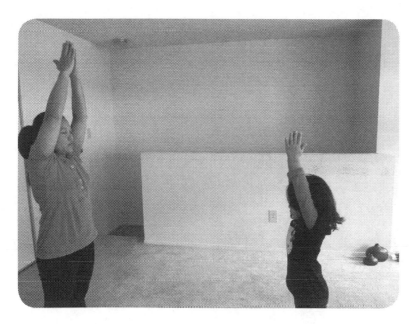

Move hands above your head in prayer pose.

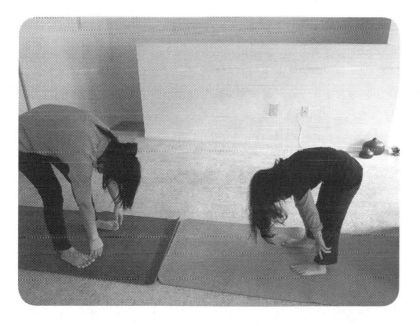

Bend down touching your toes.

Plank Pose

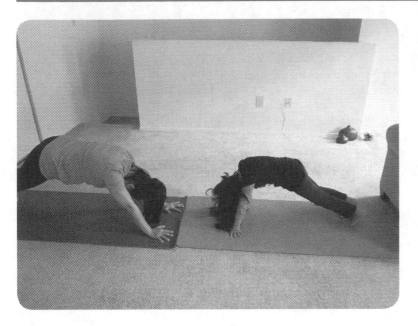

Place palms flat on the ground. Place your legs back. Push up and keep your body as straight as you can.

Cobra Pose

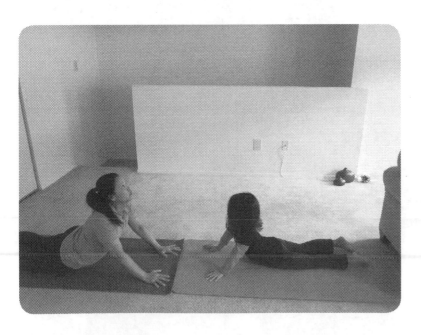

Lie on your stomach. Place your hands under your shoulders and your palms flat on the ground. Then push your chest and arms up until your arms are straight. If you're not flexible you may place your elbows on the ground. Look up and don't forget to inhale and exhale.

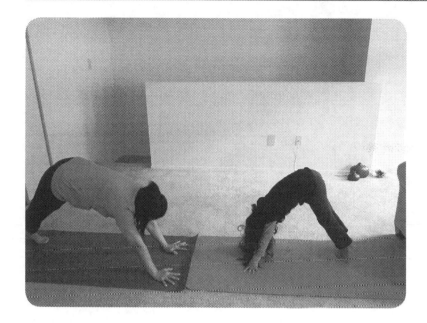

Place the palms of your hands and the soles of your feet flat on the ground. Feet are approximately hip-width apart.

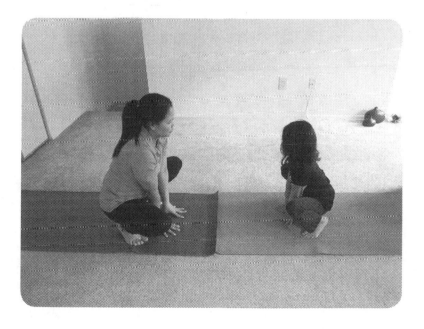

Squat down with your ankles touching and your hands on the ground.

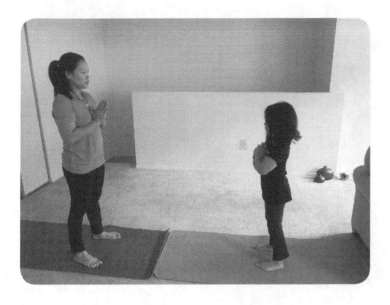

Stand with hands in prayer pose at your heart center.

Face each other throughout the Sun Salutation Series. Try to keep your eyes closed as much as possible. Repeat series 3-5 times.

After doing yoga to start her day, the daughter is very hungry. She decides that since they are in Italy they should have some pizza. The best pizzeria is in Florence. They get in a cab and go to the pizzeria.

Spinal Flex

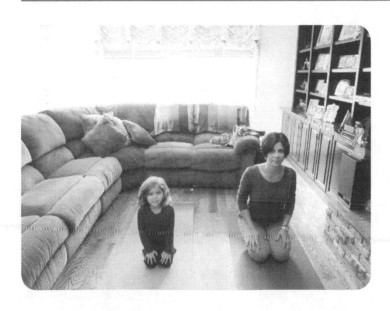

Sit on your heels in rock pose. Move your spine front and back as fast as you can with your hands on your knees. Looks like a bumpy cab ride. (1-3 minutes)

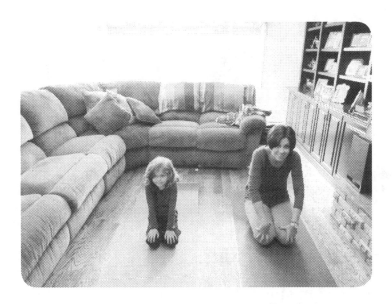

Along the way to Florence, they look out their window at the mountains of beautiful Tuscany. They also see many cats and cows.

Cat and Cow

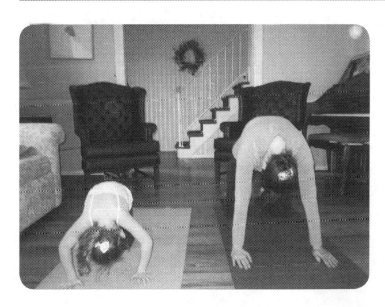

On your hands and knees inhale and arch your spine up and head down. Exhale and arch your spine down and head up. (1-3 minutes)

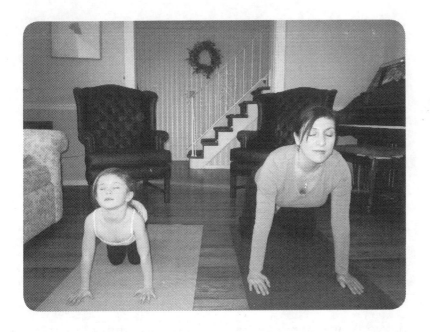

They see a cat that is so big they believe it is a lion.

Lion

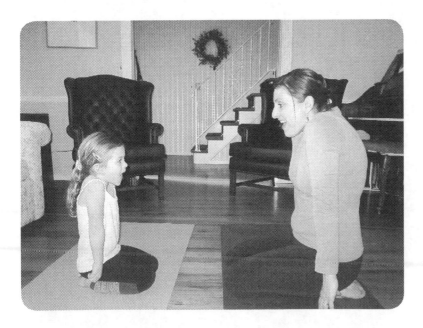

Face each other with hands by your sides. Scrunch your shoulders and roar like a lion. (1-3 minutes)

They see big trees.

Partner Tree Pose

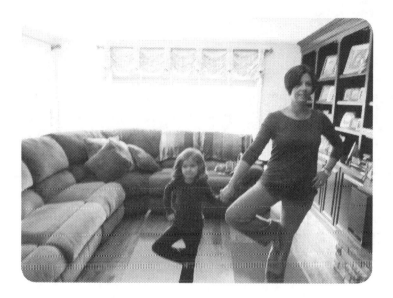

Stand on one leg with the other leg bent touching your knee or thigh. Mom and daughter hold on to each other. Change legs. It helps with balance if you find a spot and focus on it. (1-3 minutes each side)

They even see some monkeys hanging on the trees.

Monkey

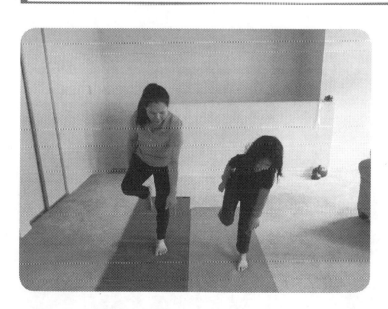

Jump up and down like a monkey. (1-3 minutes)

They finally arrive at the pizzeria in Florence. It is a small restaurant in the middle of Florence. Florence is a beautiful city. They walk into the restaurant and order a large cheese pizza because they are very hungry. The chef starts making their pie. He takes dough and tosses it in the air several times.

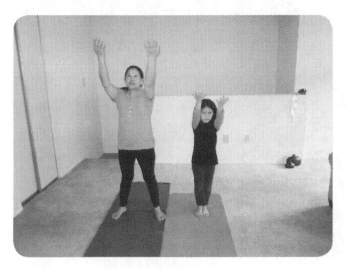

Stay standing. Touch the ground and then throw your arms up in the air. Continue doing this. It looks like rolling and throwing pizza dough in the air. (1-3 minutes)

The chef hands the baked pizza to the very hungry mom and daughter. Mom and daughter sit by the window, eat the pizza, and look at the spectacular view of Florence, Italy. Outside they see artists painting pictures of moms and daughters who are doing yoga on the street.

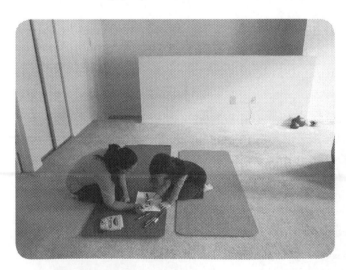

Mom and daughter together draw a picture of themselves doing a yoga pose in Italy. (5-10 minutes)

Mom and daughter love watching this. They are so happy that they hug.

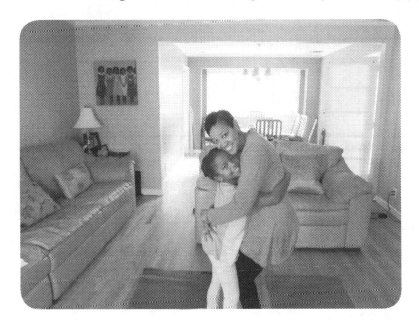

Hug

I hope the pizza was yummy! ☺

♡ Rochelle

After eating a lot of pizza in Florence, mom and daughter are very tired, so they stretch.

Stretch

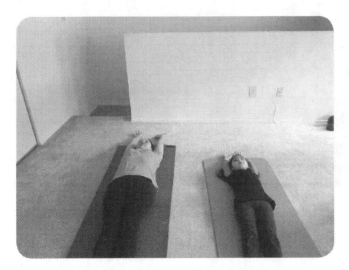

Move your arms and legs all around. (1-3 minutes)

Cat Stretch

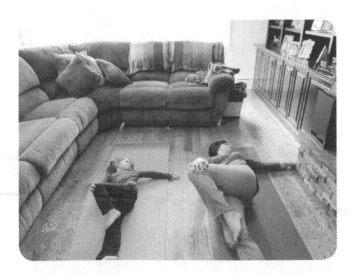

Lie on your back, bend your left knee. Put left leg over right and place your left arm out to the side. Then change to the other leg. (1-3 minutes each side)

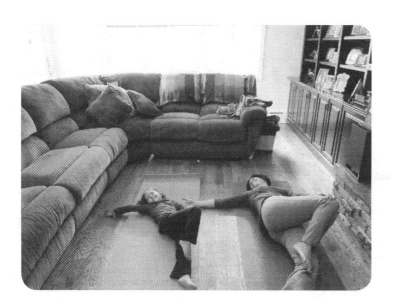

They realize that they are tired of being away from their house on Long Island, New York. They decide that they should go back to their villa, pack their bags, and go to the airport. They take a cab and return to the villa.

Spinal Flex

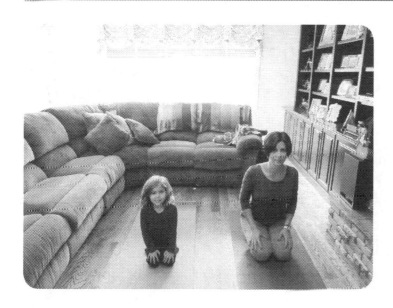

Sit on your heels in rock pose. Move your spine front and back as fast as you can with your hands on your knees. Looks like a bumpy cab ride. (1-3 minutes)

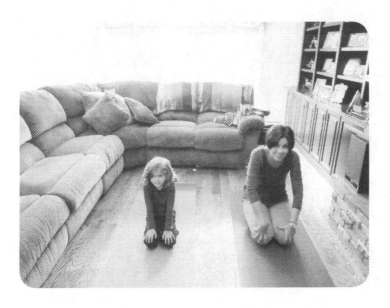

They arrive at the villa, grab their bags, and start for the airport. When they arrive at the airport, they have to buy tickets to get back to New York. They look all around to find the ticket agents.

Sufi Grind

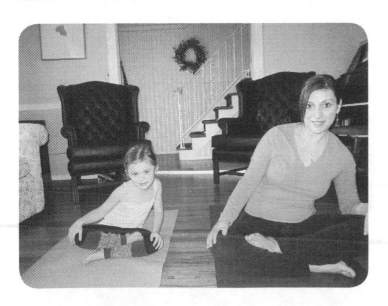

Sit in easy pose (cross-legged). Place hands on knees and move your spine all around, then change direction. (1-3 minutes each direction)

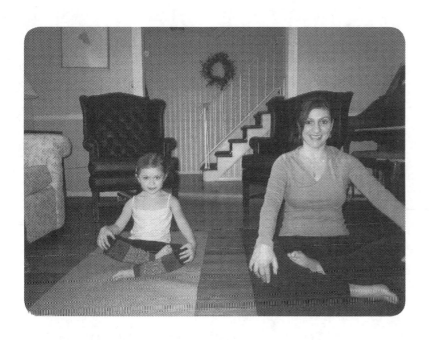

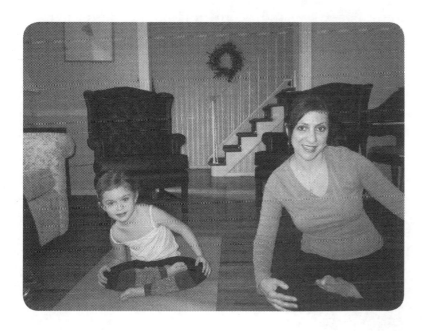

Then they look from left to right.

Spinal Twist

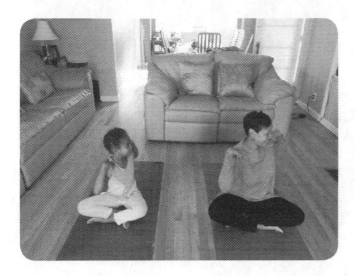

Place your hands on your shoulders
and twist from left to right.
(1-3 minutes)

At last, they find the ticket desk. Sue, a very nice lady, says that there are two tickets
to New York, but they have to transfer in Iceland. Mom and daughter agree to take
this flight. The only problem is that the plane is leaving in ten minutes. They run
to the plane.

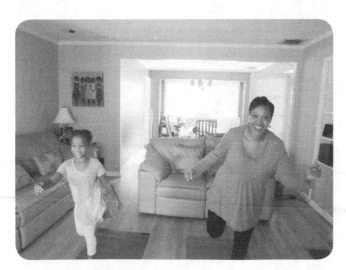

Run all around the room.
(2-3 minutes)

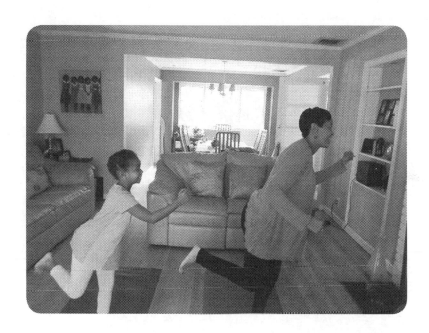

They just make it to the plane. They board the plane, and it quickly takes off.

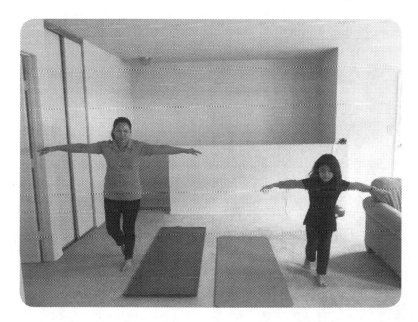

Stay standing and fly like a bird or a plane all around the room. Raise your arms very high. (1-3 minutes)

When the plane is in the air, they see beautiful clouds.

Camel Pose (Looks like a Cloud)

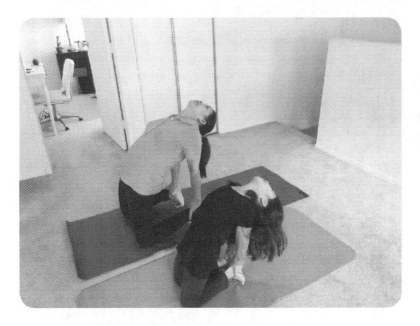

Sit on your knees, straighten your spine and lean back. Grab your ankles or heels. Adjust yourself according to your flexibility. Push the heart center upward. (1-3 minutes)

They imagine they see birds.

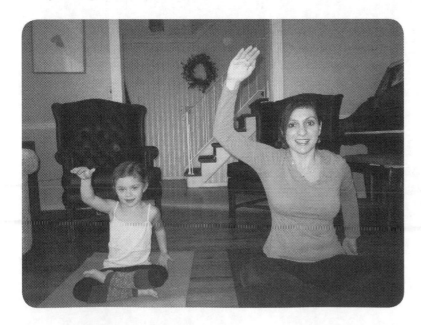

Sit in easy pose and move your arms like a bird flying. (1-3 minutes)

Then all of a sudden the plane ride starts getting bumpy.

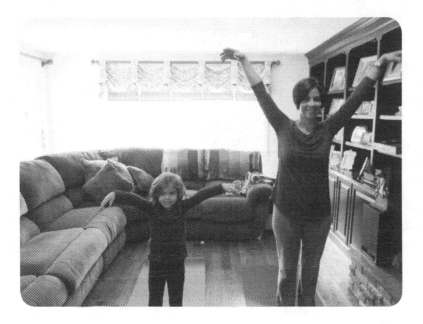

Stand up, shake, and jump. (1-3 minutes)

There must be a lot of wind outside.

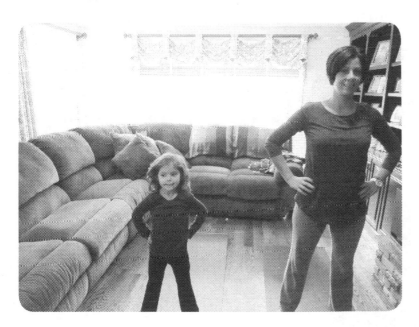

Stand hip-width apart with hands on hips and move your spine in big circles making noise that sounds like wind. (1-3 minutes)

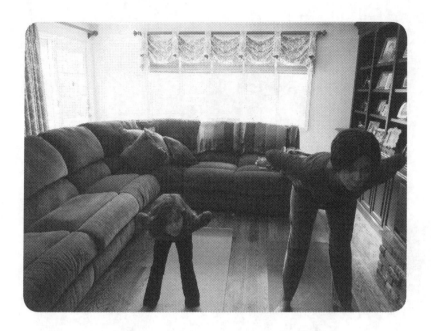

The plane is rolling from side to side.

Bundle Roll

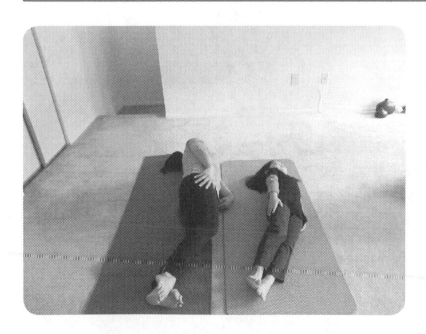

Lie down on your mat and roll to the right and then the left with your arms straight at your sides. (1-3 minutes)

Finally, the plane calms down.

Baby Pose

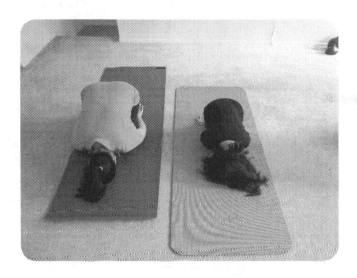

Bend forward placing your forehead on the ground. Place your third eye on the ground. The third eye is the point in between your eyebrows. Arms are at your side with palms facing up. (1-3 minutes)

Happily, they land in Iceland. They look out the window, and they see lots of snow. Now they have to take a train to the baggage claim to pick up their luggage.

Train

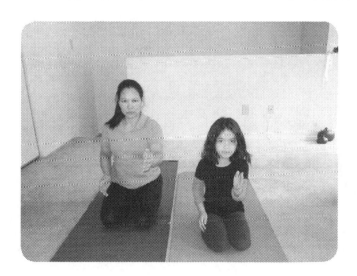

Sit in rock pose, on your heels and move your arms back and forth by your sides as fast as you can with elbows bent. Looks like a train. (1-3 minutes)

They decide to stay at a hotel near the airport because their flight to New York is the next day. When they arrive at the hotel and check into their room, they stretch.

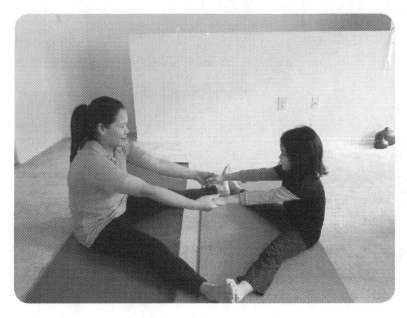

Mom and daughter get into a partner pose where the mom is seated and her legs are open really wide. The daughter either matches the mom and their feet touch or the daughter spreads her legs enough to place her feet on her mom's calves. Their hands connect, and they move back and forth really stretching the spine. (1-3 minutes; stay in this posture while the next part is read)

And they stretch some more.

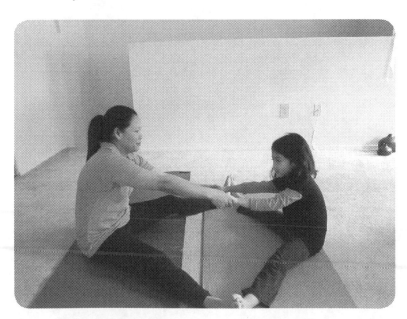

Same posture but move arms and spine around in a big circle. (1-3 minutes)

They are so happy to be off the bumpy plane that they hug.

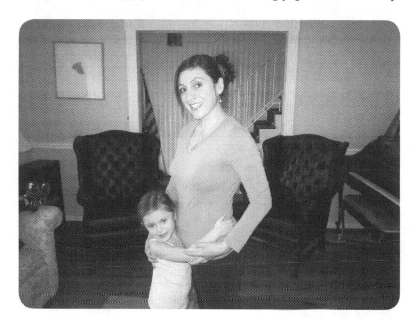

Hug

I love my mom !

♡ Rochelle

Mom and daughter arrive home from Iceland in time for Thanksgiving dinner. They are so glad to be home that they do the yoga twist.

Yoga Twist

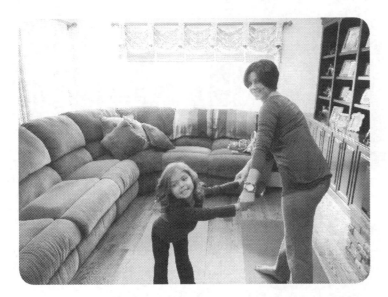

Mom and daughter face each other, hold hands, and twist in opposite directions. (1-3 minutes)

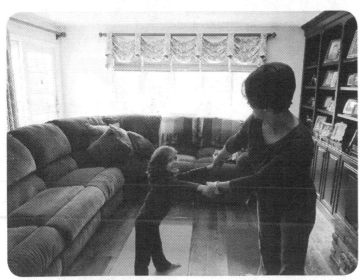

After the Thanksgiving meal they decide that they will go to the local homeless shelter and teach some yoga. That will give those less fortunate the tools to become calm and focus their minds. They begin teaching sun salutation which they recommend doing every morning to welcome the sun.

Sun Salutation Series

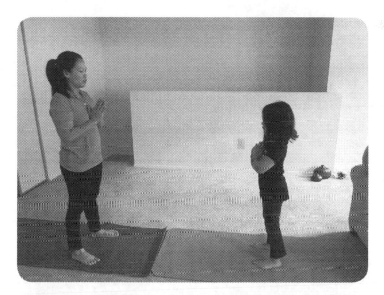

Mom and daughter arrange their mats facing each other.

Stand with hands in prayer pose at your heart center, facing each other with your eyes closed.

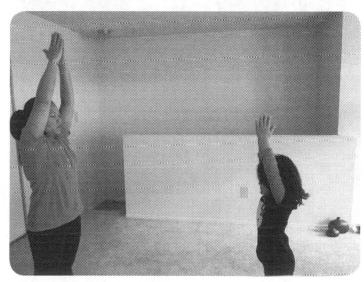

Move hands above your head in prayer pose.

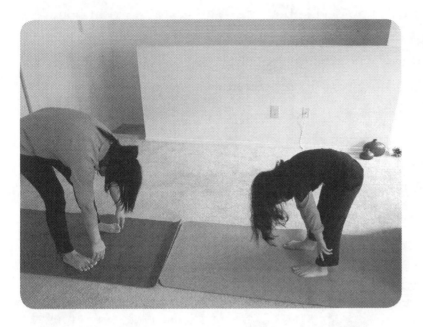

Bend down touching
your toes.

Plank Pose

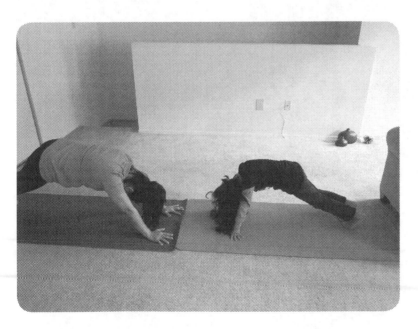

Place palms flat on the
ground. Place your legs
back. Push up and keep
your body as straight as
you can.

Cobra Pose

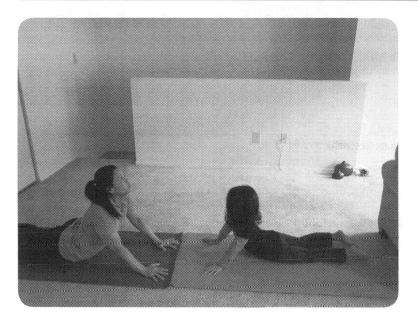

Lie on your stomach. Place your hands under your shoulders and your palms flat on the ground. Then push your chest and arms up until your arms are straight. If you're not flexible place your elbows on the ground. Look up and don't forget to inhale and exhale.

Downward Facing Dog (Triangle Pose)

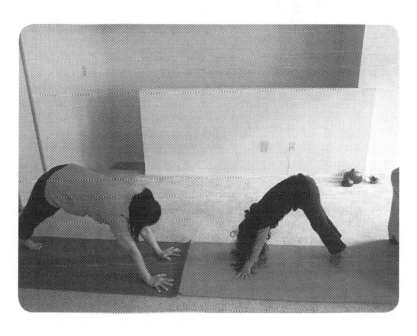

Place the palms of your hands and the soles of your feet flat on the ground. Feet are approximately hip-width apart.

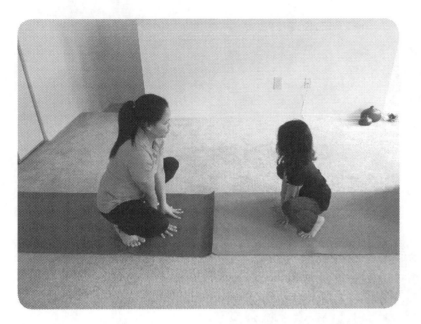

Squat down with your ankles touching and your hands on the ground.

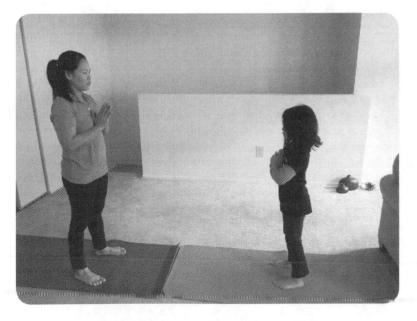

Stand with hands in prayer pose at your heart center.

Face each other throughout the Sun Salutation Series. Try to keep your eyes closed as much as possible. Repeat series 3-5 times.

Then they teach spinal exercises to give energy to help them throughout the day.

Sufi Grind

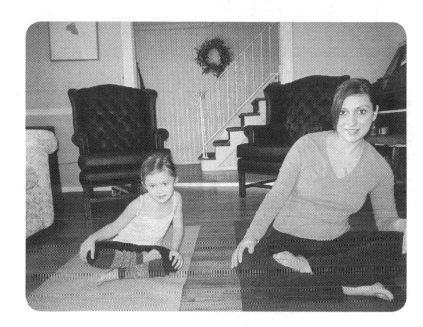

Sit in easy pose (cross-legged). Place hands on knees and move your spine all around, then change direction. (1-3 minutes each direction)

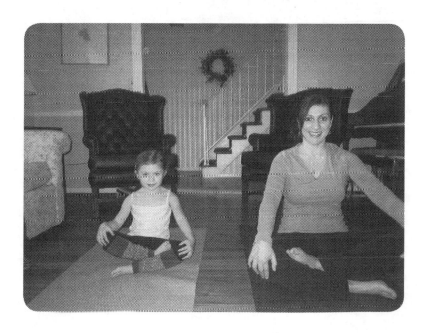

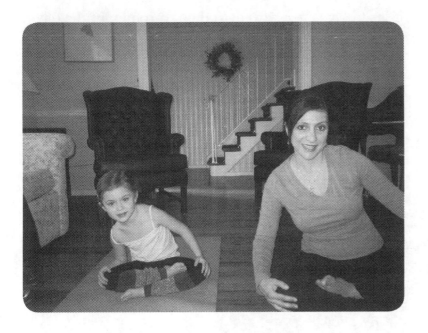

Next they look from left to right.

Spinal Twist

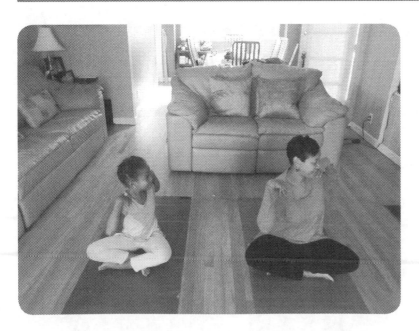

Place your hands on your shoulders and twist from left to right. (1-3 minutes)

112

When the class is finished the mom and daughter are in great moods because they helped other people. On the way home they go to the mall to see the decorations. When they arrive at the mall, they climb the stairs to go to the department store.

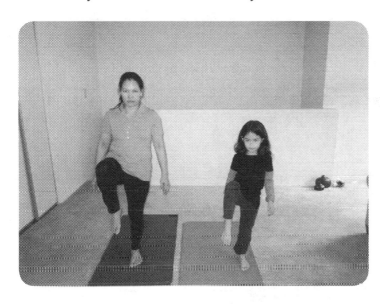

Lift legs up and down really high, like climbing stairs. (1-3 minutes)

The department store is decorated beautifully for the holidays. Mom and daughter walk all around.

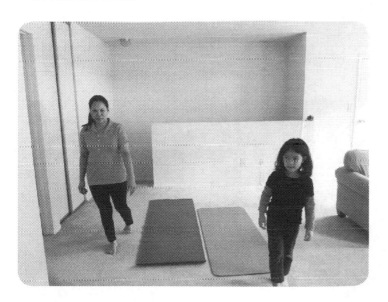

Walk all around the room. (1-3 minutes)

First, they go to the toy department where they see the prettiest rag doll. Of course, the daughter has to have it.

Rag Doll

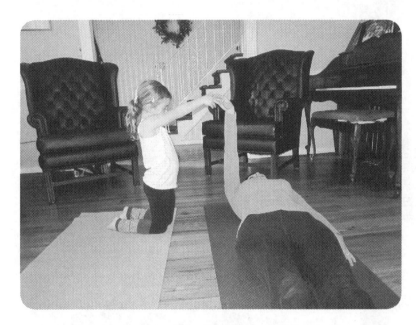

Mom lies down, and the daughter lifts mom's arms and legs. The mom has to be relaxed. Then they switch. (1-3 minutes each)

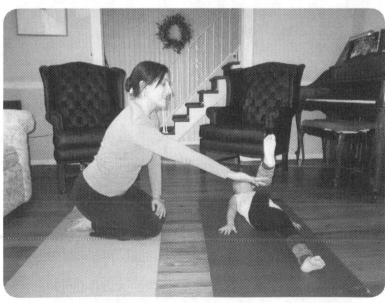

Then they continue walking. While walking around, they see women shopping with their dogs.

Downward Facing Dog (Triangle Pose)

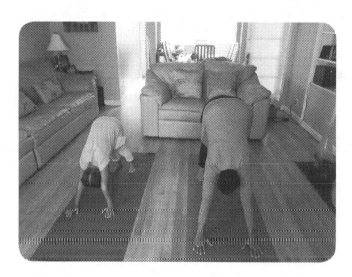

Looks like a mountain. Place the palms of your hands and the soles of your feet flat on the ground. Feet are approximately hip-width apart. (1-2 minutes)

Next they see mannequins dressed in beautiful clothes. They look as if they are doing tree pose.

Partner Tree Pose

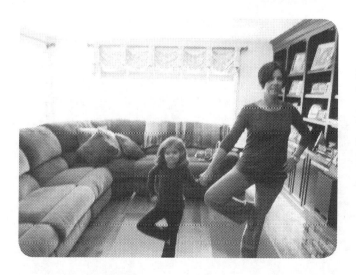

Stand on one leg with the other leg bent touching your knee or thigh. Mom and daughter hold on to each other. Change legs. It helps with balance if you find a spot and focus on it. (1-3 minutes each side)

Mom and daughter decide they will try on some clothes. They are having so much fun trying on clothes.

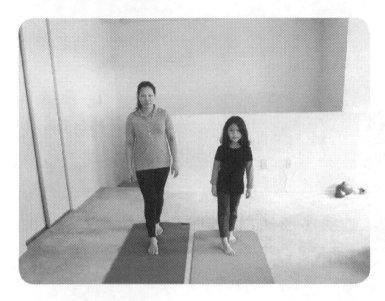

Walk back and forth on your yoga mat like a model doing the cat walk. (1-3 minutes)

Then mom and daughter become very hungry. They go to a lovely restaurant. They sit outside at this restaurant, and they see beautiful butterflies flying around.

Butterfly

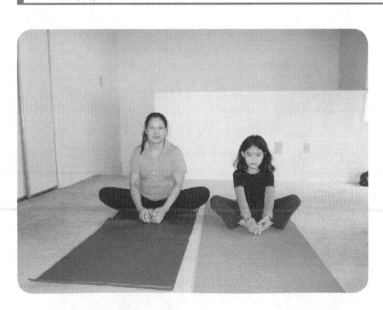

Sit in easy pose with your feet together, knees bent and move legs back and forth. Place hands on your feet. (1-3 minutes)

In addition to seeing the butterflies they look all around and see beautiful statues.

Balance Pose

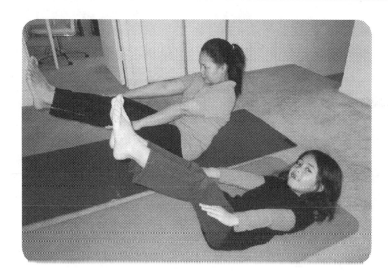

Lie on the floor. Raise your legs together 60 degrees. Lift up and place your arms out straight. (1-3 minutes)

In the middle of the outdoor restaurant, they see a lake a sunflowers. Some of the sunflowers look small and some look huge!

Seed Pose

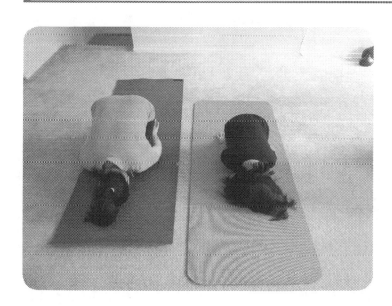

Begin in baby pose, on your heels with your stomach and head facing the ground. Bring arms back. (1 minute.)

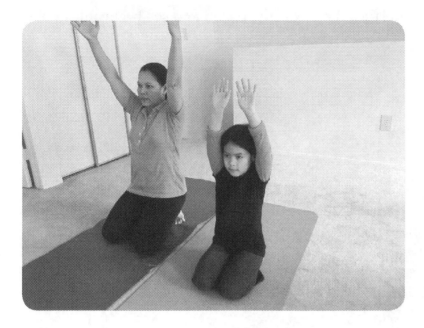

Stretch your arms up and get bigger and bigger by slowly standing up.

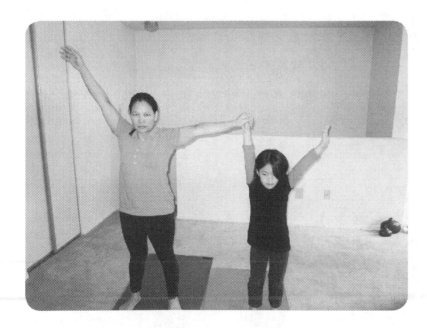

Once standing, mom and daughter grab hands and reach toward the sky. (1 minute)

They are having such a wonderful day. They are so happy that they hug.

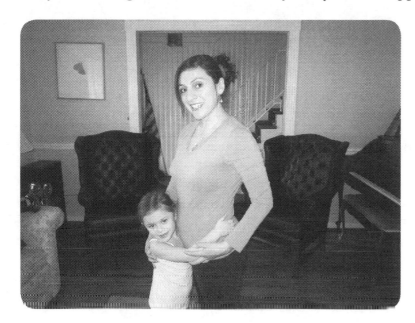

Hug

I hope you enjoyed
their adventures.

♡ Rochelle

The End for Now

Adventures of Mom and Daughter Yoga continues...

Every yoga pose listed in this book is fun and healthy. Listed below are the explanations of how these poses benefit you. Each pose is listed alphabetically. Some poses have two different names according to the different types of yoga. These names are in parentheses. Other poses have no specific yoga name. They're just great for your health!

Poses	Benefits
Archer Pose (Warrior Pose)	Brings inner strength
Baby Pose	Calms you down
Balance Pose	Great for your stomach muscles, mind and body
Bicycle Pose	Helps your legs and navel become stronger
Bridge Pose	Great for your back and legs
Bundle Roll	Reduces stress in your body
Butterfly	Opens up your hips to allow more flexibility
Camel Pose (Cloud Pose)	Helps strengthen your immune system
Cat And Cow	Allows your spine to be more flexible
Cat Stretch	Reduces stress in your back
Cat Walk	Good for the heart and brings confidence
Cobra Pose	Reduces stress in your body
Dancing	Good for your heart and a great stress reliever
Deep Relaxation	Relaxes you
Downward Facing Dog (Triangle Pose)	Good for sluggish digestion, enhances the nervous system and relaxes most of the muscle systems of the body
Fish Pose	Keeps your internal body balanced
Flying Like A Bird	Great for your arms, spine and heart
Hugging	Feels great
Lion	Great way to reduce anger
Lying Down With Mom's And Daughter's Heads Facing Each Other	Great for relaxation
Meditation Pose	Help you focus in your everyday life
Monkey Jumps	Keeps your glands functioning properly

Neck Roll	*Releases tension in your neck and helps with clear thinking*
Partner Chair Pose	*Helps flexibility in your spine and relaxes you*
Partner Rowboat	*Great for your stomach muscles and brings flexibility to your spine*
Partner Rowboat Part Two	*Great for your stomach muscles and brings flexibility to your spine*
Partner Tree Pose	*Great for your posture and helps you focus*
Rag Doll	*Great trust exercise with your partner* *Good for relaxation*
Raising Arms In The Air	*Good for your heart*

Resources

Fly Like a Butterfly by Shakta Kaur Khalsa, www.childrensyoga.com

"The Aquarian Teacher," KRI Level 1

Gratitude

I have much gratitude and wish to thank the following people......

Yogi Bhajan, his teachings have changed my life.

Shakta Kaur Khalsa, founder of the Radiant Child Yoga program <u>www.childrensyoga.com.</u> Thank you for always answering my emails and for your incredible support. *Fly Like a Butterfly* is such an inspiration to me.

Tej Kaur Khalsa, in Los Angeles, who not only came to me in a dream with words of wisdom, but who also is a dream.

Patricia Porco, owner of the best toy store, Funni Business, in Oyster Bay, Long Island. Her guidance has been unbelievable.

Joy Anne and Diana, Michele and Corinne, Angela and Sarah, Zenith and Olivia, who are the most amazing mothers and daughters! Thank you so much for agreeing to be photographed for my book. I had so much fun with all of you, and I am truly grateful for your help.

Kennie Seiz, for being extremely patient with my computer skills and for working so hard on my book. Vince, from Pantheon Entertainment, who did a great job on my yoga video and to the brilliant Jetix Design who did an incredible job on my website and everything else. To Kevin and Alex, from Glen Cove Printery, who did a wonderful job and were always willing to help me.

I thank Gail, the owner of Om Sweet Om Yoga studio, who has given me the opportunity to teach mom and daughter yoga at her beautiful studio in Port Washington, New York.

I thank Balboa Press for their patience and encouragement.

Many thanks to my wonderful, unconditionally and amazingly supportive family: my mom, dad, Uncle Michael, sister Marnie, and adorable dog Henry. Jody and Robbie but for your unbelievable support, I would be truly lost.

I also thank April, Gurmukh, Dr. Ellenmorris Tiegerman Farber, Dr. Christine Radziewicz, and Aunt Linda for your inspirational words.

I am very fortunate to have such a close, loving relationship with my own mom. She is truly my best friend and an extraordinary woman.

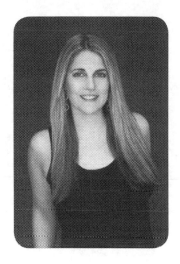

Hi, I'm Rochelle. I love yoga, and I love spending time with my mom! I am a certified yoga, prenatal yoga and children's yoga instructor. I studied under the inspirational Gurmukh Kaur Khalsa and Shakta Kaur Khalsa, who is the founder of the Radiant Child Yoga program. When I started teaching a mom and daughter yoga class, I wanted to design a yoga set for moms and daughters to do together that would be fun. So each week I wrote a story about a mom and daughter going on an adventure together that included yoga postures.

One day when I was driving—that's where I do my best thinking—I came up with the idea to put all of my stories into a book. This way not only could I help moms and daughters in my classes be healthy and get closer, but I could help moms and daughters everywhere. Another day when I was driving—again where my best thinking takes place—I came up with the idea to create a mom and daughter yoga card game and matching yoga mats. Then I had another creative moment and decided matching bracelets would be adorable. I then created My Mom's Yoga, Inc., which is where you can find me.

I hope you enjoy this book as much as I enjoyed writing it. I would love to hear from you and see how this book affected your life. Please visit me at www. MyMomsYoga.com.

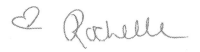

♥ ♥ ♥ *Yoga Thoughts for My Mom* ♥ ♥ ♥

♥ ♥ ♥ *Yoga Thoughts for My Daughter* ♥ ♥ ♥